Cancer and Society

Eric H. Bernicker

Editor

Cancer and Society

A Multidisciplinary Assessment
and Strategies for Action

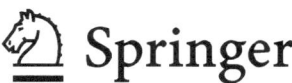 Springer

Editor
Eric H. Bernicker
Cancer Center, Houston Methodist Hospital
Houston
TX
USA

ISBN 978-3-030-05854-8   ISBN 978-3-030-05855-5   (eBook)
https://doi.org/10.1007/978-3-030-05855-5

Library of Congress Control Number: 2019932848

This Springer imprint is published by the registered company Springer Nature Switzerland AG
The registered company address is: Gewerbestrasse 11, 6330 Cham, Switzerland

Foreword

In the last decade, we have seen remarkable improvements in human health across the globe. These gains have been largely due to our successful efforts in combatting infectious diseases. With declines in deaths due to HIV, tuberculosis, malaria, and childhood diarrhea and pneumonia in every region of the world, we are seeing shifts in the global disease burden and leading causes of mortality. However, as infectious diseases retreat, the noncommunicable diseases (NCDs) are rising to take their place—including most forms of cancer. Grouping all types together, cancer is the second leading cause of death worldwide—and about half of these are considered "premature deaths" (avoidable had screening or treatment been available). This translates into about nine million deaths each year, equaling nearly one-quarter of all deaths. The majority, more than 70%, occurred in low- and middle-income countries (LMICs). And concerning trends in these countries indicate that NCDs are rising faster, affecting younger age groups, and resulting in worse outcomes.

Many factors are contributing to this alarming shift in global disease burden. First, populations in every region of the world are living longer. Currently, in low- and middle-income countries, average life expectancy is into the 60s, with an overall global average of 70 years for males and 74 years for females. A predictable consequence of this desirable trend is that, as populations age, the disease burden and distribution necessarily shift toward NCDs. Simultaneously, important changes seen in diet and lifestyle have occurred in recent years due to rapid urbanization and subsequent changes in livelihoods and social structures. As diets become more "Westernized" with more processed, high-fat foods and fewer fruits and vegetables, lifestyles become more sedentary, and the use of both tobacco and alcohol increases, it is no surprise that rates of diabetes and obesity are climbing and, along with these conditions, rates of cardiovascular disease and cancer. Lastly, infections such as hepatitis and human papilloma virus also contribute to the rise of their associated cancers, being responsible for approximately one-quarter of cancers in LMICs. Taken together, these dangerous trends are threatening our ability to reach several of the Sustainable Development Goals.

Cancer carries the additional challenge of being a heavily loaded term. It was not that long ago that people were afraid to say it out loud—even a speculative cancer diagnosis was discussed in hushed voices, behind closed doors, and often only with immediate family members, *never* with the person experiencing the disease. Even today, the word cancer instills fear and dread in the minds of most people, even those in wealthy communities who have access to comprehensive and cutting-edge treatment. In poorer communities where cancer care access is not guaranteed—either in the USA or elsewhere—the odds rarely seem to be in one's favor. Recognizing that in LMICs, 9 out of 10 patients with a cancer diagnosis will die, it is no wonder that patients wait to seek care, afraid of facing the outcome they believe is inevitable any earlier than they have to, completely unaware that earlier detection and treatment may lead to a greater chance of survival, thus reinforcing the "cancer = death sentence" paradigm.

Today our world is more connected than ever before through business, travel, and numerous social media platforms. Among other things, these connections have led to a greater recognition of the health inequities that exist across the globe. A better understanding of how cancer risk and care occurs on our currently uneven global playing field is critical for understanding the underlying issues to the growing cancer burden and why we cannot continue business as usual if we want to change the current trajectory—in this country and across the globe. In all settings, rising cancer rates will be driven by the unequal economic development that targets the poor and other historically vulnerable communities across the globe. The important influence that the social determinants of health—factors such as socioeconomic status, education level, social integration, and support systems, as well as one's physical environment and neighborhood—have on ability of individuals and populations to reach their optimal health has been well described. Those with the fewest resources and least clout will suffer the greatest negative consequences. Therefore, applying a social justice frame is necessary to best understand the factors that contribute to the uneven distribution of cancer morbidity and mortality and to inform strategies that address these multifactorial, complex health, and public health challenges.

Delving into the health equity issues associated with the current cancer burden and delivery of care and prevention services, it is tempting to focus on issues of access to cancer treatment. Clearly, this is a critical issue given that many of today's cancer medications are prohibitively expensive and therefore out of reach for most of the world's cancer patients. In fact, less than one-third of LMICs report having cancer treatment services available. Yet issues of equity extend well beyond drug prices. Access to healthcare generally and cancer screening in particular becomes relevant. And beyond health and healthcare services, the impact of broader social and environmental factors that affect cancer risk must be closely explored. These include increasing urbanization and air pollution, global changes in climate that disrupt agricultural systems and yield less nutritious food crops, and greater exposure to carcinogenic environmental toxins such as pesticides, lead, and volatile organic compounds that are the by-products of natural resource extraction—and how those living in poorer communities and nations are going to bear the brunt of these increased risks. In addition to environmental changes, consider the targeting advertising of tobacco and alcohol toward LMIC markets where the requirements for health warnings are non-existent and you have the perfect storm for the growing cancer pandemic.

Cancer care and prevention is a complex global health challenge and will require a multisectoral approach if we are going to reverse current trends or reach World Health Organization targets such as a 25% reduction in the rate of premature cancer deaths globally by 2025, along with other NCDs. Improvements in data collection and surveillance, typically in the form of comprehensive cancer registries will be necessary to help quantify the magnitude of the problem and inform national health policymakers in allocating limited resources. Replicable and scalable models of cancer care and prevention need to be shared widely with plans for broader implementation. The current situation in care and prevention is a clarion call for those of us engaged in global health to take action through advocacy, capacity building, and equity-driven research. There is no alternative if our vision is a world with health equity for all.

Lisa V. Adams
Associate Professor of Medicine
Associate Dean for Global Health
Dartmouth Geisel School of Medicine
Hanover, NH, USA

Preface

Current developments in therapeutics for cancer therapy have led to increasing optimism regarding treatment success. Developments in immunotherapy as well as rapid advances in DNA sequencing and genomics have led to an unprecedented expansion of therapeutic targets. Many patients with metastatic cancer are now going into remission and living longer than at any time in the past. While many patients do not respond to these new innovative therapy and others who do eventually develop acquired resistance, the success achieved thus far have encouraged cancer researchers that significant clinical advances will continue to accrue.

Despite these impressive scientific achievements, many public health issues that intersect directly or indirectly with cancer as a field remain problematic. Tobacco use, while much lower in the west than 40 years ago, continues to be a public health scourge in the developing world; it is estimated that tobacco will cause a billion deaths in this century. Pollution is being recognized as a growing health hazard that especially affects the health of low-income communities, especially in the global south. Access to care remains problematic in both the USA and in low- to mid-income countries. Drug expense remains an impediment to maximizing patient access, and financial toxicity remains a burden that cancer patients and their families have to shoulder, often for years following therapy. These issues both contribute to suffering of current cancer patients and often unfortunately lay the groundwork for the next generation of people who will be facing advanced malignancies.

Many oncologists and cancer researchers are more than busy focusing on their patients and narrow field of scientific investigation. However, if we take a broader view, this same group is uniquely positioned to make significant contributions to the discussion of how to best address broader issues where the field of cancer medicine overlaps with other problems facing society. Whether it is reassuring the public that the same scientific methods that have brought these significant clinical advances also are used to confirm anthropogenic climate change or continuing to lead advocacy efforts to limit tobacco use, these pressing societal problems need to be addressed by physicians on the frontline of patient care.

With aging populations, increasing documentation burden, and a well-publicized physician burnout crisis, why should healthcare professionals involve themselves in larger public health issues? Who has the time to lend their expertise and their voices to significant social issues facing society? I would argue that there are three major reasons.

Firstly, being involved in efforts to improve the public good can definitely serve as a bulwark against burnout and cynicism and infuse significant meaning that can complement the work that providers do in the lab or in the clinic.

Secondly, cancer scientists often are well regarded by the public, and they need to leverage their scientific bully pulpit, so to speak, to help inform and guide the public on the weight of evidence-based science that can inform social and political action. Whether that is discussing climate change or environmental pollution or gun control, we can bring a measured discussion of data and how to interpret it that is becoming more important and yet more elusive to our civic discourse.

Lastly, we all have a responsibility to work toward human flourishing and make sure that the future generations of life on this planet—and not just human life—can partake in the joys of living in the world. Cancer physicians and researchers understand all too well how biological systems can go awry and damage life; working to minimize tobacco or pollution or climate change is a way of limiting the damage to the biosphere and should help increase the odds of a healthy future for humanity.

This topic can be vast; we have selected only a number of pressing issues to address looking at the intersection public health and cancer as well as framing certain questions by looking at cancer patients as a vulnerable group. It is our hope that these essays will inspire oncologists and cancer researchers to occasionally look beyond the walls of the clinic and get involved—by bringing their knowledge and passion—in addressing societal issues so that we will have fewer cancer patients in future generations, not more.

Houston, TX, USA   Eric H. Bernicker

Contents

Contributors

Eric H. Bernicker, MD Thoracic Medical Oncology, Cancer Center, Houston Methodist Hospital, Houston, TX, USA

Associate Professor of Clinical Medicine, Weill Cornell Medical College, New York, NY, USA

Associate Clinical Member, Houston Methodist Research Institute, Houston, TX, USA

Houston Methodist Cancer Center, Houston, TX, USA

Mary D. Chamberlin, MD Geisel School of Medicine at Dartmouth and Norris Cotton Cancer Center, Department of Medicine and Hematology-Oncology, Lebanon, NH, USA

Yanin Chavarri-Guerra, MD, MSc Department of Hemato-Oncology, Instituto Nacional de Ciencias Médicas y Nutrición Salvador Zubirán, Tlalpan, Mexico City, Mexico

Mary K. Clancy, MSN Office of Research Protections, Houston Methodist Research Institute, Houston, TX, USA

Olivia J. Diorio, BS Department of Environmental Studies, University of Vermont, Burlington, VT, USA

Kristie L. Ebi Center for Health & the Global Environment, University of Washington, Seattle, Washington, DC, USA

Andrew M. Farach, MD Radiation Oncology, Houston Methodist Hospital, Houston, TX, USA

Jay Fitzpatrick Centre for Integrative Ecology, School of Life and Environmental Sciences, Deakin University, Geelong, Waurn Ponds, VIC, Australia

David H. Gorski, MD, PhD Department of Surgery, Wayne State University School of Medicine and the Barbara Ann Karmanos Cancer Institute, Detroit, MI, USA

Bishal Gyawali, MD, PhD Program on Regulation, Therapeutics and Law (PORTAL), Division of Pharmacoepidemiology and Pharmacoeconomics, Department of Medicine, Brigham and Women's Hospital, Harvard Medical School, Boston, MA, USA

Gilberto Lopes, MD, MBA Sylvester Comprehensive Cancer Center, University of Miami and the Miller School of Medicine, Miami, FL, USA

Nathaniel T. Matthews-Trigg Center for Health & the Global Environment, University of Washington, Seattle, Washington, DC, USA

Jens Osterkamp Department of Surgery and Transplantation, Rigshospitalet, Copenhagen Ø, Denmark

Nynke Raven Centre for Integrative Ecology, School of Life and Environmental Sciences, Deakin University, Geelong, Waurn Ponds, VIC, Australia

Bernard E. Rollin Philosophy, Colorado State University, Fort Collins, CO, USA

Megan E. Romano, MPH, PhD Geisel School of Medicine at Dartmouth and Norris Cotton Cancer Center, Department of Epidemiology and Cancer Epidemiology Research Program, Lebanon, NH, USA

Enrique Soto-Perez-de-Celis, MD, MSc Department of Geriatrics, Instituto Nacional de Ciencias Médicas y Nutrición Salvador Zubirán, Tlalpan, Mexico City, Mexico

Renee E. Stubbins, PhD Houston Methodist Cancer Center, Houston, TX, USA

Frédéric Thomas CREEC, Montpellier, France

MIVEGEC, UMR IRD/CNRS/UM 5290, Montpellier, France

Beata Ujvari Centre for Integrative Ecology, School of Life and Environmental Sciences, Deakin University, Geelong, Waurn Ponds, VIC, Australia

Jennifer Vanos School of Sustainability, Arizona State University, Tempe, AZ, USA

Haydée Cristina Verduzco-Aguirre, MD Department of Hemato-Oncology, Instituto Nacional de Ciencias Médicas y Nutrición Salvador Zubirán, Tlalpan, Mexico City, Mexico

Stephen T. C. Wong, PhD, PE Systems Medicine and Bioengineering Department, Houston Methodist Cancer Center and Houston Methodist Research Institute, Houston, TX, USA

Chapter 1
Tobacco and Social Justice

Eric H. Bernicker

Introduction

Does the world really need yet another chapter on the horrors of tobacco? It seems a little like writing a screed against slavery after the American civil war … although the effects of chattel slavery did not disappear after the guns fell silent at Appomattox and tobacco use did not cease after the American surgeon general's report of 1963. Yet given the ongoing toll that tobacco continues to take on global health (predicted to lead to over a billion deaths in the next century [1]) and the potential threats raised by the business model of big tobacco morphing to aggressively promote e-cigarettes, healthcare providers will continue to need to battle the threat to public health posed by these products.

Tobacco-related illness and suffering continue to be a major medical and economic issue in the West. However, given current trends, it is a burden that is being mostly shouldered by economically disadvantaged groups as well as vulnerable populations, such as minorities, patients with mental illness, or prisoners [2]. Current healthcare trends in America that are exacerbating healthcare disparities do not offer much hope or encouragement that tobacco control will be better funded in the future. In addition, the increasing rates of smoking in China and much of the developing world are such that a tsunami of tobacco-related deaths—not just from cancer but also strokes and pulmonary and coronary disease—is just over the horizon.

E. H. Bernicker (✉)
Thoracic Medical Oncology, Cancer Center, Houston Methodist Hospital, Houston, TX, USA

Associate Professor of Clinical Medicine, Weill Cornell Medical College, New York, NY, USA

Associate Clinical Member, Houston Methodist Research Institute, Houston, TX, USA

Houston Methodist Cancer Center, Houston, TX, USA
e-mail: Bernicker@houstonmethodist.org

© Springer Nature Switzerland AG 2019   1
E. H. Bernicker (ed.), *Cancer and Society*,
https://doi.org/10.1007/978-3-030-05855-5_1

The mechanisms of tobacco that cause carcinogenesis are well known and scientifically elucidated. Still, many smokers remain ignorant of the health risks from tobacco and often are confused about the role that nicotine plays in addiction: a confusion promoted and exploited by tobacco companies [3]. Furthermore, many physicians remain pessimistic about their ability to encourage individual patients to quit, let alone effect policy changes on a macro level. The question is whether looking at the societal problems caused by smoking through a social justice lens provides healthcare providers and activists any different vantage points for developing approaches to tackle these issues.

This chapter will briefly outline the current state of tobacco-related illness and then look at how it effects various vulnerable groups. The rise of e-cigarettes and other mechanisms of delivering nicotine will be addressed against the backdrop of an industry with a long history of deceit and obfuscation looking for new ways to profit. Lastly, we will see how looking at the global tobacco pandemic while keeping the ideas of social justice and human flourishing in mind can lead to different avenues to effect change.

While in common public discourse the term "social justice" seems vague enough to either not offend or vacuous enough to not hold actual content, in reality there are emerging and robust definitions that will serve us fruitfully here. These frameworks look not just as health functioning of individuals but at outside societal factors that impinge upon their capability to achieve flourishing [4]. From that standpoint, justice can be considered as a facilitator of human well-being [5]. "Justice," so considered, must be kept in mind by physicians, politicians, and activists as they confront products and an industry in many ways that is the iconic anti-platonic ideal of the enemy of human flourishing and the public good.

Author Rob Nixon has written eloquently of what he terms slow violence, where, because it accumulates slowly over a long period of time without the drama and visceral impact of sudden violence, can easily be missed [6]. While Nixon was writing chiefly about climate change and the dreadful implications for the poor of the world, the analogy is equally applicable to the tobacco pandemic. Indeed, the many noted correlations between Big Tobacco and Big Oil—the toxic effects of their products on human health, the denialism and attacks on science, and the power of lobbyists to prevent coordinated action for the public good—will allow us to gain important perspectives on what it will take for human flourishing to be available to a much larger percentage of the human race.

The State of Worldwide Tobacco Use and the Extent of the Problem

Tobacco has been causatively linked to multiple malignancies, such as cancer of the lung, head and neck, bladder, esophagus, liver, and colon. Beyond triggering the development of cancers, its use also has been associated with emphysema and

COPD, coronary artery disease, peripheral vascular disease, and cerebrovascular accidents. There is no safe level of tobacco use, unlike with alcohol, and the fact that it remains a legal product given the societal harm it causes raises many questions about autonomy versus communal costs.

While smoking rates have declined in many affluent Western nations, the drop seems to be levelling off [1]. Two major concerns persist regarding the different trajectories of tobacco use in the Western world and in developing countries: in the former, the major groups that continue to smoke are groups with the least access to the healthcare system, and in the latter, the use across the general population continues to rise. Approximately six million people die every year from tobacco use, and the World Health Organization estimates that there will possibly be a billion deaths in the upcoming century. Unlike other causes, such as outbreaks of infectious disease epidemics such as Ebola or influenza, these deaths are very much preventable should there be a concerted effort and will behind achieving a smoke-free world.

Tobacco deaths by the numbers are so mind-boggling and have been so often discussed that we have become numb to them. In 2015, smoking caused more than one in ten deaths worldwide, killing more than 6 million people with a global loss of nearly 150 million disability-adjusted life years [1]. Yet despite irrefutable proof that cigarettes kill smokers (as well as exposed non-smokers) and cause significant burden on public health, suggestions that these products be banned are considered wishful flights of whimsy or as an inevitable gift to criminals and smugglers destined to profit from the inevitable illegal trade. The persistent and clawing stigma that these "weak" people brought their misfortune upon themselves remains powerful and often exploited by companies who continue to insist that they are now good responsible corporate citizens who are concerned with the health of children. Yet now with ongoing massive sales expansion in lower-income nations, especially those with weak public health infrastructure, as well as the explosion in interest in e-cigarettes or heat-not-burn products, the financial future of Big Tobacco looks quite sound. Indeed, the tremendous growth of e-cigarettes might not be just a life raft for Big Tobacco but might be more akin to the new version of the iPhone, fueling new clients and product growth wrapped up in shiny technological innovation. Tobacco companies are flush with cash and seemingly well positioned to continue to market products that will turn short-term profits for them and their shareholders into death and disease with the tab being picked up by taxpayers. Many people were—and continue to be—upset that, while many banks collapsed in 2008 because of their bundling of subprime mortgage loans and needed the government to bail them out (Occupy Wall Street), similarly Big Tobacco makes the profits and sows the seeds of ongoing suffering and death, the costs of which will be borne by governments and many who never smoked and never profited. Yet because of the slow violence of tobacco (which is not just slow but now mostly over the horizon and out of view of those in high-income nations), the needed outrage of the public is not mobilized. (Why is there not an Occupy North Carolina?)

The Legal Realm

In an ironic twist, companies that manufacture medical devices or drugs—with profit in mind but with actual clinical utility at heart—often seem much more liable to damages from legal action than the tobacco companies, who clearly have no medical intent in mind with the production of their products and who have managed to shield themselves fairly successfully from ruinous penalties. There are many reasons for this, and to detail them would be beyond the scope of this article; however, years of scientific obfuscation, aggressive lobbying of legislators, and brilliant use of marketing have continued to place much of the blame for tobacco-related disease on the users rather than the manufacturers [7].

In 1998, 46 state attorneys general signed a settlement agreement with the tobacco industry called the Master Settlement Agreement (MSA). At first it seemed like a major fatal blow, taking money from the tobacco companies to offset the significant medical costs for citizens suffering from tobacco-related illness in the United States. Yet in hindsight, public health experts have not viewed the outcome favorably: the companies found ways around the advertising limitations, and much of the money that went to the states never was used for smoking education [8]. In an even more perverse twist, states now had an incentive to protect the tobacco companies as they had sold bonds based on future income from the settlement. Money that was supposed to be set aside for tobacco education was used for other purposes and state legislators not held to account [9].

Targeting Vulnerable Communities

As opposed to luxury items, marketed obviously to the rich, or food, needed by everyone, tobacco companies have pioneered marketing to the vulnerable. Future use of their products depends on either people beginning to smoke when they are children or people in disadvantaged communities who might have less access to knowledge about the truly harmful effects of tobacco. Clearly from a social justice standpoint, taking advantage of the disadvantaged should leave a fairly odious smell wafting around the industry that even menthol flavoring should be unable to hide. In the aftermath of the economic meltdown of 2008, fueled by investments in subprime mortgages, there was a plethora of ethicists questioning the ethics of predatory lending to economically disadvantaged groups. In much the same way, Big Tobacco's marketing outreach to vulnerable minority communities—especially children—has received and should continue to receive scrutiny.

It has been well documented that American children in low-income community are significantly more likely to be exposed to cigarette advertising than children in upper-scale neighborhoods [10] and for retailers to sell tobacco to them [11]. The tobacco companies learned a long time ago how advertising profoundly opened their availability to the future smokers' market—everyone remembers Joe Camel—

and while the MSA limited certain types of advertising, the omnipresent presence of convenience store tobacco signage as well as the ongoing visible ads at sporting events makes sure that the products remain visible to the next generation of smokers. Again, this is not quite akin to marketing sugary cereals to teens or hawking happy meals—products that are nutritionally suspect and harmful in large amounts but ultimately not addictive: this is marketing an addictive and often lethal product to a group, children, that society feels needs to be until they are older and have intellectually matured.

Smoking rates also remain exceptionally high among those with mental illness and prisoners (the Venn diagram of both groups would of course overlap significantly) [12, 13]. Patients with schizophrenia and depression tend to have much higher rates of smoking and to be much less able to quit. Rates of smoking in incarcerated prisoners remain high as well [13]. The irony is of course that often the continued use of tobacco in these groups is often defended on the argument that their lives are "difficult," and taking away an addictive and potentially lethal product would be cruel if it in some way decreased the quality of life of these groups. Yet common sense—as much of compassion and ethics—would suggest that prisoners and those with mental illness require greater—not less—protection from tobacco. Studies that have looked at the health benefits of making prisons tobacco-free have shown lowered mortality among prisoners with mental illness [14].

Environmental Consequences of Growing Tobacco

The societal damage wrought by tobacco is not limited to its consumption and subsequent damaging of human health, although that obviously has been the most studied and most visible. However, multiple broader issues are triggered by the growth and transport of tobacco, both in terms of the health of those who harvest the leaf and the ecological impact of tobacco farming.

Growing tobacco requires a large amount of wood for curing and building structures to store the leaf. In addition, much land needs to be cleared of trees to allow the planting of the seeds, thus tobacco farming is adding considerably to deforestation [15]. Most tobacco is now grown in developing countries, often in the highlands which are more favorable for the growth of the plant but where the ecosystem is more fragile.

Deforestation is a significant issue facing the world as anthropogenic climate change continues to grow in importance as a worldwide health issue. Besides adding to the ongoing decrease in biodiversity, deforestation affects the amount of carbon that can be sequestered from the atmosphere [16]. Thus, part of the framing of tobacco as a social justice issue needs to look at the deleterious effects that the demand for this addictive product poses for the millions of people and animals who do not smoke.

Clearly tobacco farming is not the sole driver of deforestation, but it certainly remains one of the significant drivers. Tobacco companies have downplayed the adverse effects of tobacco farming on the land and have made it difficult for farmers to diversify to crops that are more sustainable and use less land [17]. They have used green supply chains to mask the extent of their deforestation as well as hide the fact that they routinely employ child labor in low-income countries [18]. It is vital for politicians as well as advocates to continue to understand and point out that the toxic effects of cigarettes are not solely confined to people who smoke or their loved ones who are exposed to second hand smoke. The global disease burden and the costs associated with that—health expenditures for caring for those who fall ill as well as lost life-expectancy and work—also needs to include environmental damage and adding to the chances of irreversible climate change.

There are a number of other issues relatively unique to the farming of tobacco leaf that have significant health consequences. Most tobacco farms solely grow tobacco; it is well known that monoculture leads more rapidly to soil depletion and requires a much heavier use of pesticides. In addition, tobacco plants absorb nitrogen and other minerals from the soil at a much greater amount than plants harvested for food and thus require far more fertilizer. Tobacco farmers are thus exposed to two significant health risks in the course of farming: green tobacco disease and exposure to chemicals (fertilizers and pesticides).

The actual physical harvesting of the leaf itself brings significant health risks to workers. Green tobacco disease occurs when farmers absorb tobacco across their skin, especially if the leaf is wet. Symptoms include nausea, vomiting, tachycardia, and agitation. In many parts of the world where child labor is used in the tobacco fields, more vulnerable workers will be much more susceptible to the illness. As far as the pesticides, with the movement of the majority of worldwide tobacco farming to low- and middle-income countries (LMICs), many governments have much more lax laws regarding worker exposure. This exposure is actual, and the risks are not theoretical: it has been documented that tobacco farmers have evidence of DNA damage, presumably from occupational exposures to organophosphates [19].

In addition, tobacco farming in much of the world is associated with food and financial insecurity owing to the use of land for solely tobacco growing and contracts very unfavorable for workers, often strapping them with debt that leads them to hope to get out from the next season rather than switching to different crops [20].

Lastly, cigarette butts represent a major source of pollution; they are often the most common component of worldwide litter. They decompose very slowly. They add to water pollution and can make fish sick [21]. And yet very few smokers think twice about tossing a cigarette butt onto the beach or pavement through the window of their car. With the growing awareness of thirdhand smoke and the very real health issues of tobacco residue exposure, new scrutiny of the environmental effects of tobacco waste needs to be examined [22].

Often when the global societal costs of tobacco are estimated, direct health costs as well as years of life lost are examined. However, the balance sheet now must include deforestation, soil depletion, and diffusion of carcinogens and cigarette waste throughout the biosphere. Governments must hold companies responsible by making sure that companies are not passing all of these costs to society while pocketing solely the profits.

E-Cigarettes

The current explosion in the use of electronic cigarettes has led to an ongoing debate on whether these products could be a way to lead people away from tobacco or if they would be a "gateway drug" for children, capturing future clients for the industry.

Ironically, it became apparent from documents obtained from the major tobacco companies during the wave of litigation in the 1990s that industry scientists were aware of the carcinogenic effects of tobacco and some had speculated about developing a delivery system for nicotine that removed tobacco [20]. Of course at that time, these alternative products were not pursued for development as there was a concern that would amount to a recognition that cigarettes were indeed harmful and company lawyers were always thinking ahead to possible litigation. Now, these electronic cigarettes are rapidly expanding in the market. These products use solvents and heat to deliver vaporized nicotine. While in the short term, known carcinogens from tobacco are found in e-cigarette used at much lower levels compared to cigarettes, the long-term effects of inhalation over many years are unknown, and there are concerns raised in animal models that they cause DNA damage [23, 24]. What is known is that these products are effective at administering nicotine which of course is an addictive drug.

Some authorities have argued that getting smokers to switch to vaping, as using e-cigs is known, would be a positive health outcome and could lead to many people being able to quit. They point to the relatively poor success that pharmacologic therapy offers to smokers who want to stop using cigarettes and positively encourage smokers to adopt vaping. Critics point out that studies thus far have indicated that many smokers who vape also continue to use combustible cigarettes and that, more ominously, e-cigs are becoming very popular among teens—at an age where nicotine can have significant impact on their brain. In fact, some studies have shown that e-cigarettes are a gateway to later tobacco use [25]. Lastly, despite tobacco companies frequent claim that these products are certainly not for children, they continue to make flavors such as bubblegum and watermelon, no doubt to appeal to and capture the teen market and ensure a continued future client base. Vaping has become so popular in middle school that many teachers are reporting children fidgeting in class as they withdraw from nicotine and teachers' drawers are filled with confiscated e-cigs [26].

There is another issue regarding e-cigs; from a business standpoint, they provide tobacco companies with another profitable revenue stream. An argument can be made that anything that strengthens their financial position of tobacco companies is something that needs to be vigorously attacked by public health advocates. Aggressive education needs to be provided to teens that the long-term safety of these products remains unknown and that e-cigarettes are as addictive as cigarettes.

Tobacco and Ethics

Many writers, ethicists, and philosophers have worried about whether humankind's mastery of science and technology carry, alongside the amazing improvement in medicines and human comfort, the seeds of human destruction. This concern is not necessarily limited to nuclear weapons and their proliferation, as much as that subject should induce anxiety, but now includes human contribution to global warming. The burning of fossil fuels, deforestation, pollution, all stem from viewing nature as a commodity to be utilized and not protected; all are examples of a scientific materialism run amok. Many years ago, the philosopher Hans Jonas spoke of the concern he had of the unfettered advancement of human technology divorced from a sense of human responsibility toward preserving life [27]. Jonas was not a crank Luddite. But he saw clearly that human flourishing would require squaring technological advancement with an ethics of responsibility toward preserving life and nature.

The massive rise of the use of cigarettes at the turn of the last century was also fueled by technological advances. While not as impressive in some regards as the development of nuclear weapons or factory production of guns, the results have killed many more people and currently threaten even more. The production of tobacco and cigarettes that allowed easy portability and the ability to smoke anywhere facilitated the penetration of all areas of life. Manipulation of the tobacco leaf increased the nicotine content and rendered the product much more addictive. The rise of modern advertising in magazines, papers, and TV allowed the meme of glamorous smoking to penetrate the consciousness of an ever-expanding market. And with the rise of trust in science in the 1950s and 1960s, Big Tobacco used research funding and the Tobacco Institute to obfuscate and delay for as long as possible the recognition that cigarettes kill and harm. While Jonas was not thinking of cigarettes, in many ways Big Tobacco's use of technology to spread their product is the paradigm of science leading to human suffering and pollution of the environment.

So an ethics of responsibility to human flourishing would mean that healthcare workers as well as governments continue to take an uncompromising and antagonistic position against the tobacco companies. That would entail refusing to accept any funding that comes from tobacco companies. That would mean to continue to conduct rigorous research into the short- and long-term health consequences of e-cigarettes and to advocate for restrictions on sales and advertising to minors.

Lastly, healthcare workers need to become more passionately able to advocate for public health. Millennials have recently mobilized for stricter gun control laws in the wake of multiple school shootings; they also, at a number of colleges, have protested for divesting from fossil fuel companies that contribute to global warming. However, generations of activists have become numb to Rob Nixon's slow violence of tobacco; the long latency period between exposure and onset of illness coupled with the continued prominence of tobacco in movies and music has prevented the development of energetic activists and protected these multinational tobacco companies from moral scrutiny. Efforts need to continue from the medical establishment to point out that tobacco is one of the world's most lethal killers that is completely preventable and that curbing or ridding the world of tobacco would help protect not just human health but help mitigate global warming, decrease deforestation, and decrease exploitation of minorities.

Like so many medical issues that confront society, defeating tobacco and erasing the devastating health consequences is not merely one of science. Yes, we need better medications for people wanting to stop and which are more easily affordable for the poor (the cost of Chantix, a weakly effective pharmacologic approach to quitting cigarettes, is considerable and often is not well covered by insurance plans). But we also need legislative help with educating teens and limiting the reach of advertising. There are currently some signs that the FDA will attempt to decrease the amount of nicotine in cigarettes. But they also need to take a much more aggressive stance toward e-cigarette legislation and make teenagers' ability to get their hands on these products difficult. The military needs to continue to educate service men and women about the hazards of smoking and stop selling cheap cigarettes on or near military bases. Jails and psychiatric hospitals need to be strictly smoke-free and funds made available to help transition smokers off of tobacco.

The World Health Organization's Framework Convention on Tobacco Control needs ongoing support so that the shift to LMIC markets is met with improved public education in those countries. And plans must be made to help farm labor transition off of tobacco to more sustainable farming without crippling economic dislocation.

Tobacco as a cultivated and marketed product is incompatible with human health and flourishing in ways that almost all other products are not. Its continued sale is not compatible with virtually all definitions of social justice. While it is of course nonsensical to expect the complete abrogation of tobacco, there are many steps that can be taken that would make a difference. Organized medicine must take an aggressive stance against e-cigarettes for children and young adults and press for the devices to be regulated sand sold as medical devices to help smokers get off tobacco—the only defensible use of these products. Activists—for global warming, for sustainable agriculture, for preserving the environmental—need to band together and to see that the continued use of tobacco threatens all of their projects. Human rights groups that look out for vulnerable and marginalized populations need to take tobacco companies and advertisers to task.

Tobacco use is not just a medical issue—it truly is an issue that affects society at large and needs to be confronted as such. Keeping social justice concepts in mind as arguments are articulated and allies sought can hopefully help society wean off these damaging products and help envision and realize a healthier future for future generations.

References

1. Collaborators GT. Smoking prevalence and attributable disease burden in 195 countries and territories, 1990–2015: a systematic analysis from the Global Burden of Disease Study 2015. Lancet. 2017;389(10082):1885–906.
2. Grill K, Voigt K. The case for banning cigarettes. J Med Ethics. 2016;42(5):293–301.
3. Hoek J. Informed choice and the nanny state: learning from the tobacco industry. Public Health. 2015;129(8):1038–45.
4. Ruger JP. Health and social justice. New York: Oxford University Press; 2012.
5. Powers M, Faden R. Social justice: the moral foundations of public health and health policy. Oxford: Oxford University Press; 2008.

6. Nixon R. Slow violence and the environmentalism of the poor. Harvard University Press: Cambridge, MA; 2013.
7. Brandt A. The cigarette century: the rise, fall, and deadly persistence of the product that defined America. New York: Basic Books; 2009.
8. Estes J. How the big tobacco deal went bad. New York Times. 2014 Oct 6; Page A29.
9. Jayawardhana J, et al. Master Settlement Agreement (MSA) spending and tobacco control efforts. PLoS One. 2014;9(12):e114706.
10. Lee JG, et al. Inequalities in tobacco outlet density by race, ethnicity and socioeconomic status, 2012, USA: results from the ASPiRE Study. J Epidemiol Community Health. 2017;71(5):487–92.
11. Loomis BR, et al. Density of tobacco retailers and its association with sociodemographic characteristics of communities across New York. Public Health. 2013;127(4):333–8.
12. Dickerson F, et al. Cigarette smoking by patients with serious mental illness, 1999–2016: an increasing disparity. Psychiatr Serv. 2018;69(2):147–53.
13. Bailey ZD, et al. Incarceration and current tobacco smoking among black and caribbean black americans in the national survey of american life. Am J Public Health. 2015;105(11):2275–82.
14. Dickert J, et al. Decreased mortality rates of inmates with mental illness after a tobacco-free prison policy. Psychiatr Serv. 2015;66(9):975–9.
15. Geist HJ. Global assessment of deforestation related to tobacco farming. Tob Control. 1999;8(1):18–28.
16. Lawrence D, Vandecar K. Effects of tropical deforestation on climate and agriculture. Nat Clim Chang. 2015;5:27–36.
17. Benson P. Tobacco capitalism: growers, migrant workers, and the changing face of a global industry. Princeton University Press: Princeton; 2012.
18. Otañez M, Glantz SA. Social responsibility in tobacco production? Tobacco companies' use of green supply chains to obscure the real costs of tobacco farming. Tob Control. 2011;20(6):403–11.
19. Kahl VFS, et al. Chronic occupational exposure endured by tobacco farmers from Brazil and association with DNA damage. Mutagenesis. 2018;33(2):119–28.
20. Lecours N, et al. Environmental health impacts of tobacco farming: a review of the literature. Tob Control. 2012;21(2):191–6.
21. Kungskulniti N, et al. Cigarette waste in popular beaches in thailand: high densities that demand environmental action. Int J Environ Res Public Health. 2018;15(4):E630.
22. Adhami N, Chen Y, Martins-Green M. Biomarkers of disease can be detected in mice as early as 4 weeks after initiation of exposure to third-hand smoke levels equivalent to those found in homes of smokers. Clin Sci (Lond). 2017;131(19):2409–26.
23. Lee HW, et al. E-cigarette smoke damages DNA and reduces repair activity in mouse lung, heart, and bladder as well as in human lung and bladder cells. Proc Natl Acad Sci U S A. 2018;115(7):E1560–9.
24. Ratajczak A, et al. How close are we to definitively identifying the respiratory health effects of e-cigarettes? Expert Rev Respir Med. 2018;12:549.
25. Bold KW, et al. Trajectories of e-cigarette and conventional cigarette use among youth. Pediatrics. 2018;141(1):e20171832.
26. Zernike K. 'I can't stop': schools struggle with vaping explosion. New York Times. 2018 Apr 2; Page A1.
27. Jonas H. The imperative of responsibility: in search of an ethics for the technological age. Chicago: University of Chicago Press; 2000.

Chapter 2
Climate Change and Cancer

Nathaniel T. Matthews-Trigg, Jennifer Vanos, and Kristie L. Ebi

Introduction

Cancer does not come to mind when one considers the health risks of a changing climate. How might the incidence of cancer be affected by changes in temperature, precipitation, sea level rise, and increases in the frequency and intensity of extreme weather and climate events (e.g., floods, storm surges, drought, heat waves)? These changes will likely directly increase or decrease concentrations to some carcinogens and will indirectly change human behaviors that could result in increased exposure. This chapter highlights three possible pathways where climate change could alter cancer risks: exposures to particulates and carcinogenic chemicals, exposures to ultraviolet (UV) radiation, and the quantity and quality of key staples, resulting in micronutrient deficiencies.

The Intergovernmental Panel on Climate Change (IPCC) concluded that warming of the climate system is unequivocal, with many of the observed changes since the 1950s unprecedented over decades to millennia [32]. The Earth's atmosphere and ocean have warmed, the amounts of snow and ice have decreased, and sea levels have risen. In the Northern Hemisphere, 1983–2012 was likely the warmest 30-year period in the last 1400 years. Nine of the ten warmest years on record occurred since 2007 (the tenth was 1998 during an El Niño Southern Oscillation event) [91]. It is highly likely that human influence was the dominant cause of observed warming since the mid-twentieth century.

N. T. Matthews-Trigg · K. L. Ebi (✉)
Center for Health & the Global Environment, University of Washington,
Seattle, Washington, DC, USA
e-mail: krisebi@uw.edu

J. Vanos
School of Sustainability, Arizona State University, Tempe, AZ, USA

© Springer Nature Switzerland AG 2019
E. H. Bernicker (ed.), *Cancer and Society*,
https://doi.org/10.1007/978-3-030-05855-5_2

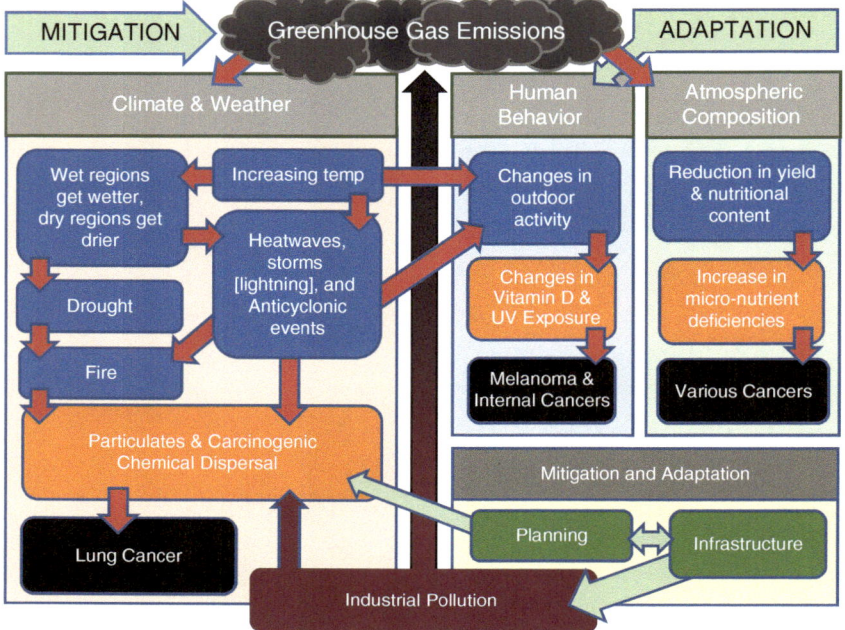

Fig. 2.1 This diagram demonstrates the complex pathways, discussed in this chapter, in which greenhouse gas emissions and resulting climate change could lead to an increase in cancers associated with air pollution, reduced nutritional intake, and UV exposure. The red arrows in the diagram signfy interaction pathways, while green arrows signify intervention opportunities

The largest contribution to these and other changes in the climate system is the increase in atmospheric concentrations of carbon dioxide (CO_2) since 1750 from burning of fossil fuels and deforestation [32]. Continued emissions of greenhouse gases (GHG) will cause further warming and changes in all components of the climate system.

Climate Change, Pollution, and Lung Cancer

Lung cancer is the leading cause of cancer mortality worldwide, causing an estimated 1.6 million deaths in 2012 [79]. The World Health Organization (WHO) estimates that 252,000 of lung cancer deaths in 2016 were attributable to air pollution. The majority of deaths were in Southeast Asia [3, 38]. The connection between exposure to fine particulate matter and lung cancer has been extensively researched, with the WHO International Agency for Research on Cancer estimating that 15% of lung cancer deaths are attributable to particulate air pollution [9, 43, 53, 57, 66, 70]. An analysis of the Global Burden of Disease found a 20%

increase in particulate air pollution deaths from 1990 to 2015 [15]. Climate change is projected to further worsen human exposure to particulate matter via complex, indirect pathways, such as increasing the risk of wildfires [1, 35, 60] and anticyclonic conditions that increase the regional concentration of anthropogenic air pollution and wildfire smoke [10, 28, 77].

Common sources of anthropogenic air pollution include vehicle exhaust, woodburning cooking stoves, emissions from power plants, manufacturing by-products, and wildfires [59]. The most significant danger is high quantities of fine particulate matter ($PM_{2.5}$: particles <2.5 microns in diameter) that can become embedded deep inside the lungs [34]. These small particles can contain carcinogens, such as polycyclic aromatic hydrocarbons (PAHs), acrolein, benzene, and formaldehyde, that can cause acute and/or chronic inflammation, thus worsening existing cardiovascular and respiratory conditions and increasing the risk of lung cancer [2, 13, 37, 68]. Anthropogenic air pollution is expected to decrease overtime as energy production and consumption practices change. The magnitude that this transition could increase UV radiation exposure and radiative forcing should be further studied. Until this transition happens, the anticyclonic conditions that exacerbate human exposure to harmful PM and ozone air pollution are projected to increase, as are the conditions that increase human exposure to wildfire smoke [22, 31] (Fig. 2.2).

Major contributing sources of greenhouse gas emissions—the drivers of climate change, such as the extraction and burning processes of fossil fuels—are greater sources of carcinogenic PAHs than forest fires and volcanic eruptions [82]. This source contribution reflects the need for local air quality regulations and global climate change mitigation efforts to reduce the health impacts of worsening wildfire smoke and industrial air pollution.

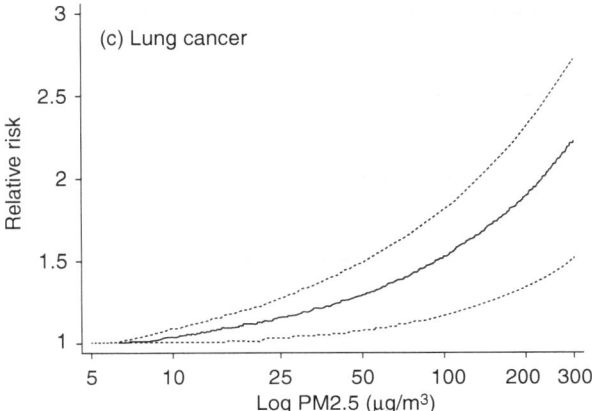

Fig. 2.2 Integrated exposure-response model of relative risk for lung cancer deaths (shaded area: 95% confidence intervals) and fine particulate (PM2.5) concentration [41]

Women in low- to middle-income countries who use solid fuels for cooking, firefighters, and low-paid workers involved in industrial manufacturing, such as aluminum, are often at greatest risk of exposure to carcinogenic air pollution [14, 30, 65].

Wildfire Smoke

Wildfires produce large quantities of carbon dioxide; $PM_{2.5}$; carcinogenic volatile organic compounds, such as benzene, formaldehyde, acrolein, and PAHs; and thousands of additional compounds [58, 71]. The connections between human exposure to volatile organic compounds and cancer risk are well-established [13, 62, 65].

Wildfire characteristics are dictated by human, meteorological, and environmental factors. Weather and human activities account for the majority of wildfire ignitions. The Intergovernmental Panel on Climate Change (IPCC), the leading global body that assesses the risks of climate change, concluded that there will likely be an increase in wildfire ignition as a result of increased lightning ([56, 60, 75, 86, 87]). Environmental factors, such as drought, available fuel (vegetation), temperature, and wind, are the largest determinants of area burned after ignition [8].

Climate change is also projected to significantly alter environmental factors that can exacerbate wildfires, such as shifting precipitation patterns, increasing temperatures, strengthening winds, and straining ecosystems ([23, 35, 47, 76, 88–90]). Although these effects are not geographically uniform, in aggregate wildfires are projected to increase in intensity, frequency, and duration, which increases the likelihood of catastrophic fire events, especially in regions with endemic wildfire and drought risk [64, 89, 90] (Fig. 2.3).

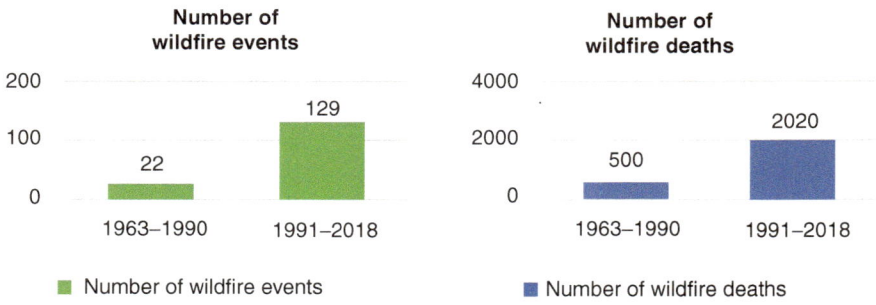

Fig. 2.3 Number of wildfire events and mortality 1963–1990 and 1991–2018. Discrepancies between 1960–1990 and 1991–2018 could be influenced by a variety of factors in addition to climate change, such as an increase in event reporting, greater human development in wildland-urban interface areas, changes in forest management practices, and others. (Reprinted with permission from Ref. [85])

Wildfires mostly impact air quality locally; however, under the right meteorological conditions, high concentrations of fine particulate matter and ozone precursor pollutants can travel large distances, increasing ground-level air pollution at regional and continental scales [49]. Recent research from Harvard projects that an additional 25 million people in the Western United States could be exposed to wildfire smoke that lasts for more than 2 consecutive days by mid-century [40]. These "smoke waves" could pose a significant risk to short-term and long-term human health, but further research is needed to understand the current and future magnitude of these impacts [39].

Climate Change and North American Western Conifer Forests

Higher temperatures and changes to precipitation patterns in the United States have contributed to the growth of endemic bark beetle populations that have killed tens of millions of trees. Various species of North American bark beetles feed on weakened or dead conifer trees, with drought-stressed or fire-weakened trees being particularly susceptible to infestation [52]. The beetles reproduce in the spring when the temperatures are warming and die off in the fall and winter when the temperatures drop. However, warmer winter temperatures from climate change cause the beetles to reproduce earlier in the year, allowing for larger populations that can cover greater distances and experience less significant die-offs in fall and winter months [48]. Although uncertainty remains about whether bark beetle-infested forests are more prone to wildfires, [76] the combined influence of climate change on wildfires and bark beetle populations has already had, and will continue to have, a dramatic impact on Western US forests and the people whose lives are connected to these forests [24] (Fig. 2.4).

Fig. 2.4 Beetle-killed trees in Colorado's Never Summer Mountains near Gould. (Source: [26])

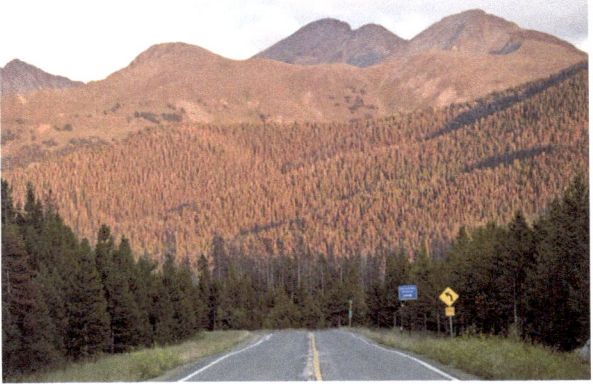

Inversions and Anthropogenic Air Pollution

Climate change is projected to increase the prevalence of anticyclonic meteorologi-cal conditions called inversions, which trap local air pollution in high-pressure domes of stagnant air [20]. These systems can move slowly or linger in place for days to weeks. Inversions dramatically increase the concentration of particulate matter and, paired with particularly toxic pollution, can cause a significant increase in morbidity and mortality if occurring over densely populated areas [5]. The mag-nitude of alteration to these anticyclonic high-pressure systems due to climate change remains uncertain due to the complexities of attribution and regional meteo-rological and geological characteristics and warrants further study [81, 90].

The danger posed by anticyclonic events, which can occur throughout the year, are largely dictated by regional anthropogenic air pollution sources and/or accom-panying high temperatures and clear skies (providing solar radiation for photo-chemical processes). If the air quality is poor, these events can pose significant dangers to people living with acute or chronic respiratory diseases, such as asthma [73]. The long-term attributable consequences of exposure to high levels of air pol-lution during a single event are difficult to ascertain; however, recent studies of the 1952 winter inversion smog event in London, UK, have demonstrated long-term health consequences [6].

Climate Change, Ultraviolet Radiation Exposure, and Skin Cancer

The projected increases in damaging UV radiation due to stratospheric ozone-depleting substances have been largely prevented due to the Montreal Protocol. However, complexities arise at the intersection of UV radiation, climate change, and stratospheric ozone that can result in benefits and risks to humans. The net effect of changes in ozone concentrations and temperature in the upper and lowest strato-sphere is complex, and additional factors such as changes in GHG emissions and cloud cover will play a vital role in model projections of future UV levels reaching Earths' surface [78]. Models project that by 2100, clear sky UV radiation and thus erythemal UV (UV_{ery}) will have increased slightly in the tropics, decreased slightly in the midlatitudes, and decreased considerably at the poles [4, 46]. However, the magnitude of projected changes in UV_{ery} differs by region and will be largely influ-enced by changes in cloud cover and aerosols in the second half of the century (whereas the first half is controlled by ozone layer recovery) [4, 46].

The reduction of anthropogenic aerosols to improve air quality is potentially the most significant factor (yet most uncertain) in increasing UV radiation reaching Earth's surface [4, 78], particularly in heavy populated areas that currently have high amounts of particulate pollution. For example, expected reductions of aerosols over the most populated areas of the Northern Hemisphere may result in 10–20% increases in UV_{ery} (even larger increases are projected over China) [4].

The major health benefit of exposure to UV_{ery} is the production of vitamin D for providing crucial support for bone metabolism, with new evidence of protection against other internal cancers (e.g., colorectal cancer, breast cancer), yet these protective effects remain largely inconclusive [51]. However, it is difficult to provide messaging regarding "safe" and "unsafe" exposures to sunlight due to interpersonal variability and location, thus pointing toward more personalized monitoring approaches to determine personal dose and response.

Although projections of UV radiation reaching Earth's surface are sparse and complex, human time-activity patterns and behavior related to sun protection are perhaps the most difficult parameters to predict, yet variations in these parameters are also the most critical to understand for the prevention of skin cancers [25, 33, 36]. Demographic and behavioral risk factors for sunburns include being a younger adult (e.g., 18–29 years of age) and engaging in more versus less physical activity [29]. Changes in weather patterns due to climate change could alter time-activity patterns and thus the prevalence of sun exposures and skin cancers. People living in areas expected to experience warmer, drier conditions have an increased tendency to spend more time outdoors [7], yet when temperatures reach uncomfortable levels, time outside may start to decline. Hence, increasing temperatures and heat waves may cause sun avoidance and act as a protective factor in southern regions for some individuals.

Alternatively, in cooler regions experiencing earlier and warmer springs, fair weather invites people to spend more time outdoors, thereby increasing exposure to UV if sunscreen use and other preventive actions (e.g., time spent in full sun vs. in shade) are not taken. However, the increased sun exposure may also reduce vitamin D deficiency in high latitudes. This behavior would be expected to markedly increase personal UV exposure in northern latitudes [78], with potentially greater impacts in low-income populations with less ability to implement sun protection [16]. Increasing temperatures and heat waves could increase sun avoidance based on risk factor guidance and thermal comfort [27]. Finally, a direct effect of climate change on skin temperature risk has been shown through increased skin carcinogenesis with temperature and humidity [21]. Values correspond to an increase of the effective UV dose by 2% for every °C rise in ambient temperature, yet the exact nature of the correlation with temperature requires further studies [72].

An improved awareness by health providers and public health agencies concerning how climate change could alter the risks of skin cancers by region is needed to ensure that preventive measures are timely and effective. Current climate-skin cancer models assume that the personal dose of UV radiation is a constant fraction of ambient UV radiation in all years and across all regions [19, 78], which is well-known to differ across individuals and regions. Increased ground level and personal monitoring via devices and apps (e.g., [36, 45, 63, 74]) are also needed to understand time-activity patterns as they relate to region and weather. The ability to accurately quantify personal UV exposures can inform effective behavior interventions, particularly for those at most risk (fair-skinned, children) to prevent an increase in skin cancers. Although uncertainty exists in future behavior and exposure, it is likely that behavior associated with climate change mitigation, rather than ozone depletion, may be a larger determinant in UV exposures and consequently skin cancer [18].

Cancer and Changes in the Quality
and Quantity of Important Stable Crops

Climate change is affecting food security [54]. Increasing temperatures, changes in the hydrologic cycle, and increases in the frequency and intensity of extreme weather and climate events (e.g., floods, droughts, and heat waves) are altering the yields of cereal crops that remain the world's most important sources of food, including wheat, rice, and maize, with further changes projected as the climate continues to change (Fig. 2.5) [11]. In tropical and temperate regions, without additional efforts to reduce impacts, climate change will negatively affect production for local temperature increases of 2 °C, although individual locations may benefit [54].

In addition, climate change will affect the nutritional quality of wheat, rice, and other staples [42]. The elemental chemical composition of a plant (e.g., ionome) reflects a balance between carbon, obtained through atmospheric CO_2, and the remaining nutrients, obtained from the soil. Higher concentrations of CO_2 stimulate plant photosynthesis and growth. However, over a hundred individual studies and several meta-analyses concluded that projected increases in atmospheric CO_2 can result in an ionomic imbalance for most plant species, with carbon increasing disproportionally to soil-based nutrients [42, 50, 67]. Major cereal crops, particularly rice and wheat, and tubers, such as potatoes, respond to higher CO_2 by increasing synthesis of carbohydrates (e.g., starches and sugars) to the detriment of protein and by reducing the quantity of minerals, such as iron and zinc [42] (Fig. 2.6).

The nitrogen decline with higher CO_2 concentrations also results in a decline in B vitamins [84]. A recent experiment conducted in China and Japan of 18 of the most common strains of rice grown under atmospheric CO_2 concentrations expected by the end of the twenty-first century resulted in a 10.3% reduction in protein and significant reductions in iron (8% less) and zinc (5.1% less) when compared with rice grown under current CO_2 concentrations. In addition, vitamin B1 (thiamine) levels decreased by 17.1%, vitamin B2 (riboflavin) by 16.6%, vitamin B5 (pantothenic acid) by 12.7%, and vitamin B9 (folate) by 30.3%. The resulting nutritional deficits are likely to hit hardest in countries where rice makes up a major portion of daily diets. The only vitamin to increase was vitamin E (tocopherol).

Therefore, climate change will result in tropical and some temperate regions producing lower yields staple crops, with those crops of lower nutritional quality. Together, these could affect susceptibility to and the incidence of various cancers. The B vitamins are involved in multiple cellular mechanisms that could influence the risks of some cancers. For example, riboflavin deficiency may increase the risk of some cancers such as breast cancer [61, 80]. Higher folate intake is associated with lower incidence of colorectal, esophageal, and pancreatic cancers [44, 69, 83]. Further, maternal consumption of specific food groups comprising "healthy" items of the Mediterranean diet, preconception use of folic acid, and intake of vitamins during pregnancy were associated with decreased risk of acute lymphocytic leukemia in their children [17].

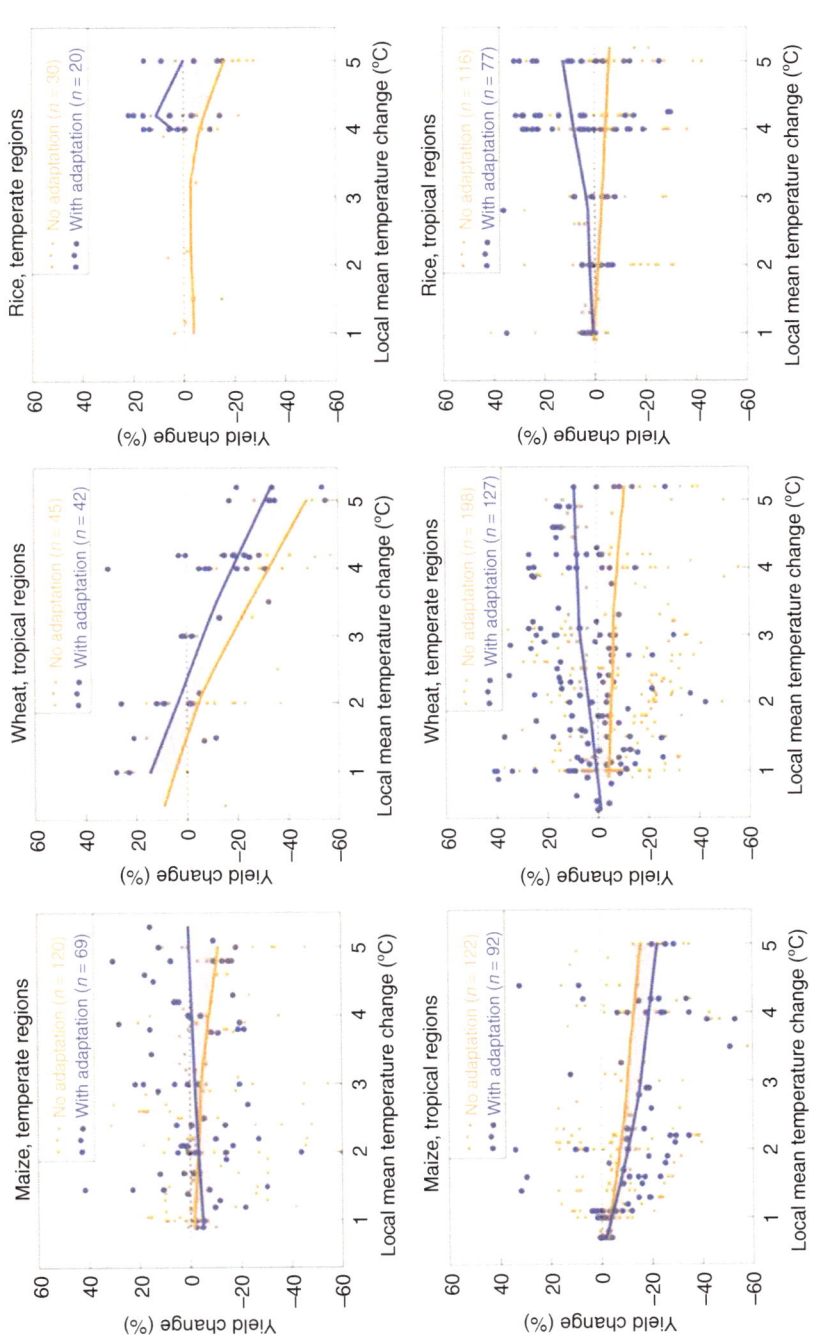

Fig. 2.5 Percent change in yield for maize, wheat, and rice as a function of local temperature change with climate change, for temperate and tropical regions, with and without adaptation. (Source: [11])

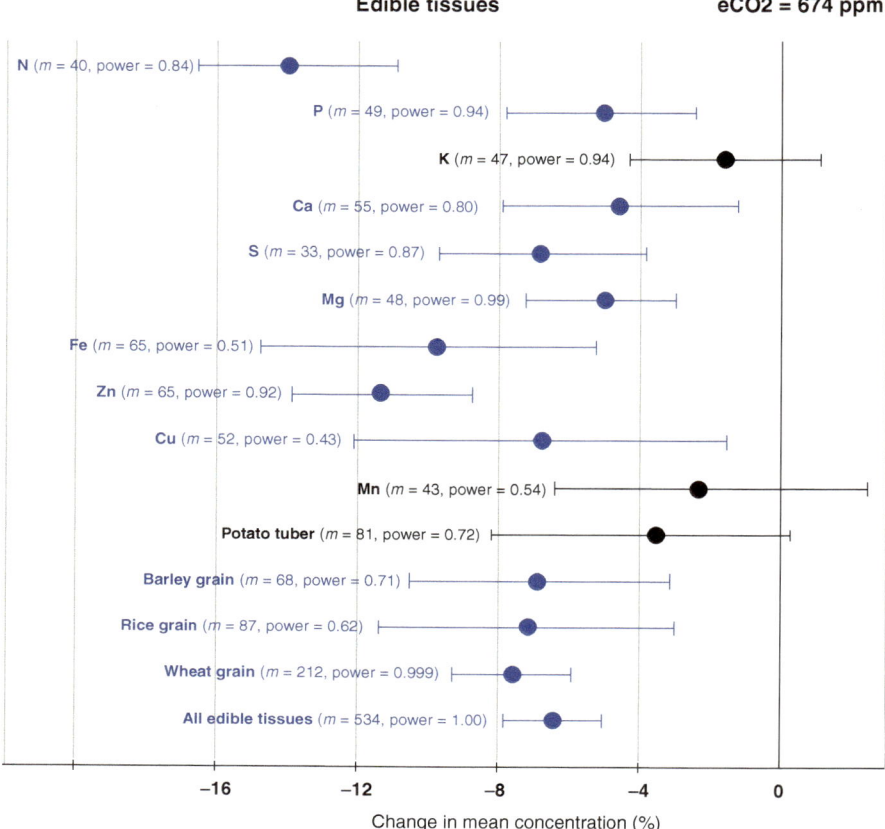

Fig. 2.6 Change (%) in the mean concentration of chemical elements in edible tissues of crops grown at CO2 concentrations expected later in the century, relative to ambient concentrations. (Source: [42])

More than 300 enzymes and more than 1000 transcription factors require zinc for their activities [55]. Lower serum concentrations of zinc also are implicated in the incidence of several cancers, including breast, gallbladder, lung, colon, health neck, and bronchus [12].

Conclusions

As illustrated in the three examples, changing weather patterns and behaviors associated with a changing climate will likely increase exposure to a range of carcinogens and/or decrease protective factors. The literature in this area is nascent, with significant knowledge gaps that, when filled, will provide a more comprehensive picture of how the incidence of cancer could change with climate change and of effective adaptation and mitigation options to reduce the additional risks to the extent possible.

References

1. Abatzoglou JT, Williams AP. Impact of anthropogenic climate change on wildfire across western US forests. Proc Natl Acad Sci. 2016;113:11770–5. https://doi.org/10.1073/pnas.1607171113.
2. Abdel-Shafy HI, Mansour MSM. A review on polycyclic aromatic hydrocarbons: source, environmental impact, effect on human health and remediation. Egypt J Pet. 2016;25:107–23. https://doi.org/10.1016/J.EJPE.2015.03.011.
3. Ambient (outdoor) air quality and health: key facts. (n.d.) http://www.who.int/news-room/fact-sheets/detail/ambient-(outdoor)-air-quality-and-health
4. Bais AF, McKenzie RL, Bernhard G, Aucamp PJ, Ilyas M, Madronich S, Tourpali K. Ozone depletion and climate change: impacts on UV radiation. Photochem Photobiol Sci. 2015;14(1):19–52.
5. Bell ML, Davis DL. Reassessment of the Lethal London Fog of 1952: novel indicators of acute and chronic consequences of acute exposure to air pollution. Environ Health Perspect. 2001;109:389–94. https://doi.org/10.2307/3434786.
6. Bharadwaj P, Zivin JG, Mullins JT, Neidell M. Early-life exposure to the great smog of 1952 and the development of asthma. Am J Respir Crit Care Med. 2016;194:1475–82. https://doi.org/10.1164/rccm.201603-0451OC.
7. Bharath AK, Turner RJ. Impact of climate change on skin cancer. J R Soc Med. 2009;102(6):215–8.
8. Bradstock R, Hammill KA, Collins L, Price O. Effects of weather, fuel and terrain on fire severity in topographically diverse landscapes of South-Eastern Australia. Landscape Ecol. 2009; 25(4):607–19. https://doi.org/10.1007/s10980-009-9443-8.
9. Brook D, Cromar K, De Matteis S, et al. A joint ERS/ATS policy statement: what constitutes an adverse health effect of air pollution? An analytical framework. Eur Respir J. 2017;49:1–34. https://doi.org/10.1183/13993003.00419-2016.A.
10. Caserini S, Giani P, Cacciamani C, et al. Influence of climate change on the frequency of daytime temperature inversions and stagnation events in the Po Valley: historical trend and future projections. Atmos Res. 2017;184:15–23. https://doi.org/10.1016/J.ATMOSRES.2016.09.018.
11. Challinor AJ, Watson J, Lobell DB, Howden SM, Smith DR, Chhetri N. A meta-analysis of crop yield under climate change and adaptation. Nat Clim Chang. 2014;4:287–91. https://doi.org/10.1038/NCLIMATE2153.
12. Chasapis CT, Loutsidou AC, Spiliopoulou CA, Stefanidou ME. Zinc and human nutrition: an update. Arch Toxicol. 2012;86:521–34.
13. Chen S-C, Liao C-M. Health risk assessment on human exposed to environmental polycyclic aromatic hydrocarbons pollution sources. Sci Total Environ. 2006;366:112–23. https://doi.org/10.1016/j.scitotenv.2005.08.047.
14. Choi H, Harrison R, Komulainen H, et al. Polycyclic aromatic hydrocarbons. In: WHO guidelines for indoor air quality: selected pollutants. Geneva: World Health Organization; 2010.. https://www.ncbi.nlm.nih.gov/books/NBK138709/.
15. Cohen AJ, Brauer M, Burnett R, et al. Estimates and 25-year trends of the global burden of disease attributable to ambient air pollution: an analysis of data from the Global Burden of Diseases Study 2015. Lancet. 2017;389:1907–18. https://doi.org/10.1016/S0140-6736(17)30505-6.
16. Dadlani C, Orlow SJ. Planning for a brighter future: a review of sun protection and barriers to behavioral change in children and adolescents. Dermatol Online J. 2008;14(9):1.

17. Dessypris N, Karalexi MA, Ntouvelis E, Diamantaras AA, Papadakis V, Baka M, et al. Association of maternal and index child's diet with subsequent leukemia risk: a systematic review and meta analysis. Cancer Epidemiol. 2017;47:64–75.
18. Diffey B. Climate change, ozone depletion and the impact on ultraviolet exposure of human skin. Phys Med Biol. 2003;49(1):R1.
19. Dijk A, Slaper H, den Outer PN, Morgenstern O, Braesicke P, Pyle JA, Garny H, Stenke A, Dameris M, Kazantzidis A, Tourpali K. Skin cancer risks avoided by the Montreal Protocol—worldwide modeling integrating coupled climate-chemistry models with a risk model for UV. Photochem Photobiol. 2013;89(1):234–46.
20. Gramsch E, Cáceres D, Oyola P, et al. Influence of surface and subsidence thermal inversion on PM2.5 and black carbon concentration. Atmos Environ. 2014;98:290–8. https://doi.org/10.1016/j.atmosenv.2014.08.066
21. de Gruijl FR, Forbes PD. UV-induced skin cancer in a hairless mouse model. BioEssays. 1995;17(7):651–60. https://doi.org/10.1002/bies.950170711.
22. Fann N, Brennan T, Dolwick P, et al. Ch. 3: air quality impacts. In: The impacts of climate change on human health in the United States: a scientific assessment. Washington, DC: U.S. Global Change Research Program; 2016. p. 69–98.
23. Flannigan M, Stocks B, Wotton B. Climate change and forest fires. Sci Total Environ. 2000;262:221–9. https://doi.org/10.1016/S0048-9697(00)00524-6.
24. Gibson K, Negron JF. Fire and bark beetle interactions. The Western Bark Beetle Research Group: A Unique collaboration with Forest Health Protection, Proceedings of a symposium at the 2007 Society of American Foresters Conference, US Forest Service, Pacific Northwest Research Station, PNW-GTR-784. 2009;51–70.
25. Godar DE. UV doses of American children and adolescents. Photochem Photobiol. 2001;74(6):787–93.
26. Greer K, USDA Forest Service (2012). Bark beetle kill leads to more severe fires, right? Well, maybe. Accessed June 2018. https://www.hcn.org/issues/44.8/bark-beetle-kill-leads-to-bigger-fires-right-well-maybe
27. Hajat S, O'Connor M, Kosatsky T. Health effects of hot weather: from awareness of risk factors to effective health protection. Lancet. 2010;375(9717):856–63.
28. He C, Wu B, Zou L, Zhou T. Responses of the summertime subtropical anticyclones to global warming. J Clim. 2017;30:6465–79. https://doi.org/10.1175/JCLI-D-16-0529.1.
29. Holman DM, Berkowitz Z, Guy GP, Hartman AM, Perna FM. The association between demographic and behavioral characteristics and sunburn among US adults—National Health Interview Survey, 2010. Prev Med. 2014;63:6–12.
30. International Agency for Research on Cancer Working Group on the Evaluation of Carcinogenic Risk to Humans (2012) Chemical agents and related occupations. Monographs on the evaluation of Carcinogenic Risks to Humans, No. 100F. https://www.ncbi.nlm.nih.gov/books/NBK304404/
31. IPCC. Climate change 2014: Synthesis Report. Contribution of Working Groups I, II and III to the Fifth Assessment Report of the Intergovernmental Panel on Climate Change, R.K. Pachauri and L.A. Meyer, eds., IPCC, Geneva. 2014;151.
32. IPCC. Summary for policymakers. In: Stocker TF, Qin D, Plattner G-K, Tignor M, Allen SK, Boschung J, Nauels A, Xia Y, Bex V, Midgley PM, editors. Climate change 2013: the physical science basis. Contribution of Working Group I to the Fifth Assessment Report of the Intergovernmental Panel on Climate Change. Cambridge/New York: Cambridge University Press. 2013;28.
33. Italia N, Rehfuess EA. Is the Global Solar UV Index an effective instrument for promoting sun protection? A systematic review. Health Educ Res. 2011;27(2):200–13.
34. Jang A-S. Particulate air pollutants and respiratory diseases. Air Pollut Compr Perspect. 2012:153–74. https://doi.org/10.5772/51363.
35. Jin Y, Goulden M, Faivre S, et al. Identification of two distinct fire regimes in southern California: implications for economic impact and future change. Environ Res Lett. 2015;10:094005. https://doi.org/10.1088/1748-9326/10/9/094005.

36. Køster B, Søndergaard J, Nielsen JB, Allen M, Bjerregaard M, Olsen A, Bentzen J. Feasibility of smartphone diaries and personal dosimeters to quantitatively study exposure to ultraviolet radiation in a small national sample. Photodermatol Photoimmunol Photomed. 2015;31(5):252–60.
37. Li X, Yang Y, Xu X, et al. Air pollution from polycyclic aromatic hydrocarbons generated by human activities and their health effects in China. J Clean Prod. 2016;112:1360–7. https://doi.org/10.1016/J.JCLEPRO.2015.05.077.
38. Lim SS, Vos T, Flaxman AD, et al. A comparative risk assessment of burden of disease and injury attributable to 67 risk factors and risk factor clusters in 21 regions, 1990–2010: a systematic analysis for the Global Burden of Disease Study 2010. Lancet. 2012;380:2224–60.. [PubMed: 23245609]
39. Liu JC, Pereira G, Uhl SA, et al. A systematic review of the physical health impacts from non-occupational exposure to wildfire smoke. Environ Res. 2015;136:120–32. https://doi.org/10.1016/j.envres.2014.10.015.
40. Liu JC, Mickley LJ, Sulprizio MP, et al. Particulate air pollution from wildfires in the Western US under climatic change (2016). Climate Change. 2016;138:655. https://doi.org/10.1007/s10584-016-1762-6.
41. Lo WC, Shie RH, Chan CC, Lin HH. Burden of disease attributable to ambient fine particulate matter exposure in Taiwan. J Formos Med Assoc. 2017;116:32–40.
42. Loladze I. Hidden shift of the ionome of plants exposed to elevated CO_2 depletes minerals at the base of human nutrition. eLife. 2014;3:02245. https://doi.org/10.7554/eLife.02245.
43. Loomis D, Huang W, Chen G. The International Agency for Research on Cancer (IARC) evaluation of the carcinogenicity of outdoor air pollution: focus on China. Chin J Cancer. 2014;33:189–96. https://doi.org/10.5732/cjc.014.10028.
44. Mason JB, Tang SY. Folate status and colorectal cancer risk: a 2016 update. Mol Asp Med. 2017;53:73–9.
45. McKenzie R. UV radiation in the melanoma capital of the world: what makes New Zealand so different?. In AIP Conference Proceedings 2017 Feb 22 (Vol. 1810, No. 1, p. 020003). AIP Publishing.
46. McKenzie RL, Aucamp PJ, Bais AF, Björn LO, Ilyas M, Madronich S. Ozone depletion and climate change: impacts on UV radiation. Photochem Photobiol Sci. 2011;10(2):182–98.
47. Mike F, Brian S, Merritt T, Mike W. Impacts of climate change on fire activity and fire management in the circumboreal forest. Glob Chang Biol. 2009;15:549–60. https://doi.org/10.1111/j.1365-2486.2008.01660.x.
48. Mitton JB, Ferrenberg SM, Benkman NHECW. Mountain pine beetle develops an unprecedented summer generation in response to climate warming. Am Nat. 2012;179:E163–71. https://doi.org/10.1086/665007.
49. Munoz-Alpizar R, Pavlovic R, Moran MD, et al. Multi-year (2013-2016) PM2.5wildfire pollution exposure over North America as determined from operational air quality forecasts. Atmosphere (Basel). 2017;8 https://doi.org/10.3390/atmos8090179.
50. Myers SS, Zanobetti A, Kloog I, Huybers P, Leakey ADB, Bloom A, et al. Rising CO_2 threatens human nutrition. Nature. 2014;510:139–42.
51. Norval M, Lucas RM, Cullen AP, De Gruijl FR, Longstreth J, Takizawa Y, Van Der Leun JC. The human health effects of ozone depletion and interactions with climate change. Photochem Photobiol Sci. 2011;10(2):199–225.
52. Parker TJ, Clancy KM, Mathiasen RL. Interactions among fire, insects and pathogens in coniferous forests of the interior western United States and Canada. Thomas J. Parker. 2006; Agricultural and Forest Entomology - Wiley InterScience. Agric For Entomol. 2006;8:167–89. https://doi.org/10.1111/j.1461-9563.2006.00305.x.
53. Pope CA, Burnett RT, Thun MJ, et al. Lung cancer, cardiopulmonary mortality, and long-term exposure to fine particulate air pollution. JAMA. 2002;287:1132–41. https://doi.org/10.1001/jama.287.9.1132.
54. Porter JR, Xie L, Challinor AJ, Cochrane K, Howden SM, Iqbal MM, Lobell DB, Travasso MI. Food security and food production systems. In: Field CB, Barros VR, Dokken DJ, Mach KJ, Mastrandrea MD, Bilir TE, Chatterjee M, Ebi KL, Estrada YO, Genova RC, Girma B,

Kissel ES, Levy AN, MacCracken S, Mastrandrea PR, White LL, editors. Climate change 2014: impacts, adaptation, and vulnerability. Part A: global and sectoral aspects. Contribution of Working Group II to the Fifth Assessment Report of the Intergovernmental Panel on Climate Change. Cambridge/New York: Cambridge University Press; 2014. p. 485–533.

55. Prasad AS. Discovery of human zinc deficiency: its impact on human health and disease. Adv Nutr. 2013;4:176–90.

56. Price CDR. Possible implications of global climate change on global lightning distributions and frequencies. J Geophys Res Atmos. 2018;99:10823–31. https://doi.org/10.1029/94JD00019.

57. Raaschou-Nielsen O, Andersen ZJ, Beelen R, et al. Air pollution and lung cancer incidence in 17 European cohorts: prospective analyses from the European study of cohorts for air pollution effects (ESCAPE). Lancet Oncol. 2013;14:813–22. https://doi.org/10.1016/S1470-2045(13)70279-1.

58. Ramesh A, Hood D, Guo Z, Loganathan B. Global Environmental Distribution and Human Health Effects of Polycyclic Aromatic Hydrocarbons. Global Contamination Trends of Persistent Organic Chemicals. CRC Press, Taylor & Francis Group. 2012;1:97–128. https://doi.org/10.1201/b11098-7.

59. Ravindra K, Sokhi R, Van Grieken R. Atmospheric polycyclic aromatic hydrocarbons: source attribution, emission factors and regulation. Elsevier Ltd, Netherlands. Atmos Environ. 2008;42:2895–921. https://doi.org/10.1016/J.ATMOSENV.2007.12.010.

60. Romps DM, Seeley JT, Vollaro D, Molinari J (2014) Projected increase in lightning strikes in the United States due to global warming. Science (80-) 346:851 LP-854.

61. Saedisomeolia A, Ashoori M. Riboflavin in human health: a review of current evidences. Adv Food Nutr Res. 2018;83:57–81.

62. Schoeny R, Poirier K (1993). Provisional guidance for quantitative risk assessment of poly cyclic aromatic hydrocarbons. U.S. Environmental Protection Agency, Office of Research and Development, Office of Health and Environmental Assessment, Washington, DC, EPA/600/R-93/089 (NTIS PB94116571).

63. Shi Y, Manco M, Moyal D, Huppert G, Araki H, Banks A, Sen-Gupta E. Soft, stretchable, epidermal sensor with integrated electronics and photochemistry for measuring personal UV exposures. PLoS One. 2018;13(1):e0190233.

64. Spracklen DV, Mickley LJ, Logan JA, et al. Impacts of climate change from 2000 to 2050 on wildfire activity and carbonaceous aerosol concentrations in the western United States. J Geophys Res Atmos. 2009;114 https://doi.org/10.1029/2008JD010966.

65. Stec AA, Dickens KE, Salden M, et al. Occupational exposure to polycyclic aromatic hydrocarbons and elevated cancer incidence in firefighters. Sci Rep. 2018;8:2476. https://doi.org/10.1038/s41598-018-20616-6.

66. Straif K, Cohen A, Samet JM, et al (2013). Air pollution and cancer. International Agency for Research on Cancer Scientific Publication No. 161. https://www.iarc.fr/en/publica tions/books/sp161/AirPollutionandCancer161.pdf

67. Taub DR, Miller B, Allen H. Effects of elevated CO2 on the protein concentration of food crops: a meta-analysis. Glob Chang Biol. 2008;14:565–75.

68. Technical Support Document EPA's 2011 National-scale Air Toxics Assessment (2011). NATA:14. https://www.epa.gov/sites/production/files/2015-12/documents/2011-nata-tsd.pdf.

69. Tio M, Andrici J, Cox MR, Eslick GD. Folate intake and the risks of upper gastrointestinal cancers: a systematic review and meta-analysis. J Gastroenterol Hepatol. 2014;29:250–8.

70. Turner MC, Krewski D, Pope CA, et al. Long-term ambient fine particulate matter air pollution and lung cancer in a large cohort of never-smokers. Am J Respir Crit Care Med. 2011;184:1374–81. https://doi.org/10.1164/rccm.201106-1011OC.

71. Urbanski SP, Hao WM, Baker S. Chapter 4 chemical composition of wildland fire emissions. Dev Environ Sci. 2008;8:79–107. https://doi.org/10.1016/S1474-8177(08)00004-1.

72. van der Leun JC, Piacentini RD, de Gruijl FR. Climate change and human skin cancer. Photochem Photobiol Sci. 2008;7(6):730–3.

73. Vanos JK, Cakmak S, Kalkstein LS, Yagouti A. Association of weather and air pollution interactions on daily mortality in 12 Canadian cities. Air Qual Atmos Health. 2015;8:307–20. https://doi.org/10.1007/s11869-014-0266-7.

74. Vanos JK, McKercher GR, Naughton K, Lochbaum M. Schoolyard shade and sun exposure: assessment of personal monitoring during Children's physical activity. Photochem Photobiol. 2017;93(4):1123–32.
75. Veraverbeke S, Rogers BM, Goulden ML, et al. Lightning as a major driver of recent large fire years in North American boreal forests. Nat Clim Chang. 2017;7:529.
76. Westerling AL, Hidalgo HG, Cayan DR, Swetnam TW. Warming and earlier spring increase Western U.S. forest wildfire activity. Science. 2006;313:940–3. https://doi.org/10.1126/science.1128834.
77. Wilbanks TJ, Romero P, Lankao M, et al. In: Parry ML, Canziani OF, Palutikof PJ, et al., editors. Industry, settlement and society. Climate change 2007: impacts, adaptation and vulnerability. Contribution of Working Group II to the Fourth Assessment Report of the Intergovernmental Panel on Climate Change. Cambridge: Cambridge University Press; 2007. p. 357–90.
78. Williamson CE, Zepp RG, Lucas RM, Madronich S, Austin AT, Ballaré CL, Norval M, Sulzberger B, Bais AF, McKenzie RL, Robinson SA. Solar ultraviolet radiation in a changing climate. Nat Clim Chang. 2014;4(6):434.
79. Wong MCS, Lao XQ, Ho K-F, et al. Incidence and mortality of lung cancer: global trends and association with socioeconomic status. Sci Rep. 2017;7:14300. https://doi.org/10.1038/s41598-017-14513-7.
80. Yu L, Tan Y, Zhu L. Dietary vitamin B2 intake and breast cancer risk: a systematic review and meta-analysis. Arch Gynecol Obstet. 2017;295:721–9.
81. Zhang X, Lu C, Guan Z. Weakened cyclones, intensified anticyclones and recent extreme cold winter weather events in Eurasia. Environ Res Lett. 2012;7 https://doi.org/10.1088/1748-9326/7/4/044044.
82. Zhang Y, Tao S. Global atmospheric emission inventory of polycyclic aromatic hydrocarbons (PAHs) for 2004. Atmos Environ. 2009;43:812–9. https://doi.org/10.1016/J.ATMOSENV.2008.10.050.
83. Zhao Y, Guo C, Hu H, Zheng L, Ma J, Jiang L, et al. Folate intake, serum folate levels and esophageal cancer risk: an overall and dose-response meta-analysis. Oncotarget. 2017;8:10458–69.
84. Zhu C, Kobayashi K, Loladze I, Zhu J, Jiang Q, Xu X, et al. Carbon dioxide (CO_2) levels this century will alter the protein, micronutrients, and vitamin content of rice grains with potential health consequences for the poorest rice-dependent countries. Sci Adv. 2018;4:eaaq1012.
85. Guha-Sapir D, Hoyois PH, Wallemacq P, Below R. Annual disaster statistical review 2016: the numbers and trends. Brussels: CRED; 2016.
86. Price C, Rind D. Possible implications of global climate change on global lightning distributions and frequencies. J. Geophys. Res. 1994;99:10823–31. https://doi.org/10.1029/94JD00019
87. Goldammer JG, Price C. Potential impacts of climate change on fire regimes in the tropics based on magicc and a GISS GCM-Derived lightning model. Kluwer Academic Publishers. Climatic Change. 1998;39:273. https://doi.org/10.1023/A:1005371923658
88. Littell JS, McKenzie D, Peterson DL, and Westerling AL. Climate and wildfire area burned in western U.S. ecoprovinces, 1916–2003. Ecol Appl. 2009;19:1003–1021. https://doi.org/10.1890/07-1183.1
89. Flannigan M, Stocks B, Turetsky M, Wotton, M. Impacts of climate change on fire activity and fire management in the circumboreal forest. Global Change Biol. 2009;15:549–560. https://doi.org/10.1111/j.1365-2486.2008.01660.x.
90. IPCC. Climate Change 2007: Impacts, Adaptation and Vulnerability. Contribution of Working Group II to the Fourth Assessment Report of the Intergovernmental Panel on Climate Change. Parry ML, Canziani OF, Palutikof JP, van der Linden P, Hanson CE eds. Cambridge University Press. 2007.
91. Climate Central. The 10 Hottest Global Years on Record. 2018. http://www.climatecentral.org/gallery/graphics/the-10-hottest-global-years-on-record.

Chapter 3
Pollution, Cancer Risk, and Vulnerable Populations

Megan E. Romano, Olivia J. Diorio, and Mary D. Chamberlin

Introduction

Cancer is no longer a problem just for wealthier countries. Statistics from GLOBOCAN 2012 suggest that more than half of cancer patients reside in developing countries and a far greater proportion of these patients die compared to those in developed countries due to limited health-care infrastructure for early detection and treatment of cancer [1–3]. The burden of cancer in low-income countries is most likely far worse than these numbers indicate as data collection is limited and tumor registries are largely absent. Many patients go undiagnosed and uncounted resulting in an unclear representation of the issue at hand.

There are also emerging differences in biologic behavior in certain cancer diagnoses. Cancers appear at younger ages than in developed countries and have more aggressive behavior. This often leads to earlier metastases and death, the reasons for which are not yet clear. Environmental pressures such as chronic infections and pollution are possible etiologies for these differences. In this chapter we will highlight the impact of pollution on the economically vulnerable as a potentially preventable cause of cancer and present two focus studies on populations in Ecuador and Rwanda.

M. E. Romano
Geisel School of Medicine at Dartmouth and Norris Cotton Cancer Center, Department of Epidemiology and Cancer Epidemiology Research Program, Lebanon, NH, USA

O. J. Diorio
Department of Environmental Studies, University of Vermont, Burlington, VT, USA

M. D. Chamberlin (✉)
Geisel School of Medicine at Dartmouth and Norris Cotton Cancer Center, Department of Medicine and Hematology-Oncology, Lebanon, NH, USA
e-mail: Mary.D.Chamberlin@hitchcock.org

© Springer Nature Switzerland AG 2019
E. H. Bernicker (ed.), *Cancer and Society*,
https://doi.org/10.1007/978-3-030-05855-5_3

Vulnerable Populations and Cancer Prevention

In the context of public health, a group of people within a larger community who experience a disproportionately high risk of adverse health outcomes, including premature mortality, comprise a vulnerable population [4]. Poverty, neighborhood quality, nutritional status, race/ethnicity, and access to healthcare influence a wide range of health outcomes. Vulnerability is a consequence of limited access to or availability of resources relative to health status [4]. In the United States, individuals with low socioeconomic status, from minority racial and ethnic groups, or without insurance experience greater rates of cancer incidence and mortality and less frequently participate in recommended cancer screenings [5]. Cancer diagnosis and treatment present special challenges in these populations due to barriers to screening and reduced access to healthcare. Further, socioeconomic disadvantages may correspond to adverse conditions of daily life, such as food insecurity, increased hardship, or psychosocial stress, which significantly impact health and well-being [6]. Racial and ethnic minorities and economically disadvantaged individuals frequently present with a later stage of cancer diagnosis and tend to have poorer survival [7]. Within the global community, people living in low-resource countries can be broadly considered as vulnerable populations due to limited access to healthcare and higher mortality rates from conditions highly treatable in other settings.

Prioritization of and political commitment to cancer prevention and control may be lacking in low-resource settings, particularly in locations where indigenous infectious diseases pose a large risk to public health and safety. Low- and middle-income countries are estimated to contribute 80% of new cases of cervical cancer annually due in part to low vaccination rates for human papillomavirus and to challenges to screening in low-resource settings [8]. Incidence and mortality of cancers caused by infectious agents (e.g., cancer of the cervix or liver) remain high in less-developed countries while the incidence of cancers more commonly caused by environment risk factors rise [9]. Successful screening strategies require resources and infrastructure that are not easily implemented in low-resource settings. These barriers to diagnosis and care lead to an increased global burden of cancer among economically vulnerable populations, though innovative cancer screening strategies, like the one pairing community-based education with multimodal breast and cervical screening in rural Honduras [10], show promise and may prove useful for improving cancer screening practices in other low- and middle-income countries.

Environmental Justice in a Changing Chemical Landscape

Increasing levels of industrialization change the chemical backdrop of a country. When environmental protections and regulations do not keep pace, vulnerable populations are often at the greatest risk of adverse health consequences. Thus, vulnerable populations pose a special concern in the context of cancer and environmental justice. In tandem with an increased risk of cancer and cancer mortality among

economically vulnerable populations, many environmental toxicants also disproportionately affect these groups (e.g., air pollution, lead, pesticides) [11–15].
Pesticides encompass a wide array of chemicals used to kill insects, vermin, weeds,
or fungus [16]. Exposure to organochlorine pesticides [e.g., dichlorodiphenyltri-
chloroethane (DDT), hexachlorobenzene, hexachlorocyclohexane] tends to be
greater among developing versus developed countries [17]. High- and middle-
income countries produce pesticides for continued sale and marketing to low-
income countries, though some of these chemicals have been banned for use within
the producing country [18]. Protection of economically vulnerable populations
across the world from pesticides will require cooperative efforts across governments
and international borders to implement truly global bans of the most hazardous
pesticides, improve protection of workers, and promote safer pest control [19].

Pesticide Safety in Low-Resource Settings

A lack of knowledge about the dangers of pesticides contributes to adverse health
consequences of pesticide exposure, as does an inability to access proper supplies
and disposal streams. A substantial knowledge base exists related to safe use of
pesticides, including the use of proper personal protective equipment (PPE), techniques for safely mixing pesticides, procedures for storage and disposal, clean-up
and hygiene practices to reduce exposure to workers and their families, and restricted
entry intervals designed to prevent pesticide exposure to workers returning to the
fields following application [20]. Many industrialized countries require training,
licensing, and access to proper equipment for pesticide workers, but developing
countries often lack these worker protections [19]. Communities surrounding agricultural operations are exposed to pesticides through spray drift, polluted water, and
soil contamination related to inappropriate disposal of pesticides [19]. Researchers
in Ghana have reported unsafe handling practices, such as using hands to mix pesticides, determining if the pesticide mix is correct by tasting it, or using inappropriate spraying tools [21–23]. In Ethiopia, pesticide safety education is uncommon
among workers [24, 25], and many farmers report having never used PPE [26, 27].
Storage of pesticides within the domicile or reuse of containers for food or water
storage, homes in close proximity to spraying activities, and lack of access to washing facilities also increase pesticide exposure for families of agricultural workers
[19]. A survey of coffee and cotton farms in Tanzania revealed pesticide containers
with missing labels or no mixing instructions and hazardous storage of pesticides in
close proximity to food or fires [28]. Old or improper equipment, complex labels
coupled with poor literacy, shortage of safe disposal options, inappropriate combination of products or use of products on the wrong crop type (e.g., cotton pesticides
on produce), and lack of sufficient national regulations are common themes leading
to increased pesticide exposure across low-resource countries [19]. These observations collectively underscore the critical need for pesticide safety education and
regulation to protect economically vulnerable communities from both cancer and
non-cancer health consequences of agricultural pesticides.

Pesticide Exposure and Cancer Risk Among Farmers, Families, and Children

Particularly among agricultural workers, the epidemiologic literature broadly supports associations between pesticide exposure and several types of cancer, including non-Hodgkin lymphoma, multiple myeloma, leukemia, brain, prostate, pancreas, breast, colon/rectum, kidney, and lung [29, 30]. Though workers tend to be at the greatest risk given their higher cumulative exposures to pesticides, research also suggests that living in an area of high pesticide use increases risk of several cancer types even for individuals not directly involved in agricultural activities [31]. Certain groups, including the developing fetus, infants, children, and older adults, are especially vulnerable to the effects of toxicants in the environment [32]. It is estimated that women in developing countries produce 60–80% of food and comprise more than 40% of the global agricultural workforce [19, 33]; thus pesticide exposure during the reproductive years is likely. A study based in Spain observed suggestive trends of increasing concentrations of placental organochlorine pesticides, such as DDT, with lower occupational social class [14], illustrating that even during pregnancy, economically vulnerable women may have increased risk of pesticide exposure. Hematopoietic and central nervous system cancers in childhood have been linked to early-life pesticide exposure [34]. A study based in Brazil suggested that the children of women exposed to pesticides during pregnancy were twice as likely to develop acute lymphoid leukemia and five times as likely to develop acute myeloid leukemia before reaching 1 year of age compared to children of unexposed mothers. Even stronger associations were observed among children of mothers exposed specifically to organophosphate pesticides or with mothers engaged in agricultural work during pregnancy [35]. A meta-analysis of 16 case-control studies further suggests that exposure to indoor insecticides corresponds to a 47% increased risk of leukemia and a 43% increased risk of lymphoma during childhood [36]. Preliminary research has indicated that in addition to prenatal pesticide exposure, preconception exposure to pesticides by either parent may lead to increases in childhood brain tumors [37], underscoring the need to protect agricultural workers and economically vulnerable populations from pesticide exposure.

Focus on Ecuador: Working Through Sociopolitical Barriers to Treat Cancer Amidst a Battle Over Oil and Biodiversity in Ecuador's Amazon

Since the discovery of oil in Yasuni National Park, Ecuador, in 1964, there has been relatively little attention paid to the effects of oil pollution on the plants, ecosystem, and indigenous communities of the Amazon. The oil contamination brought on by deliberately cheap and out-of-date technology used for extraction has been taking place for four decades, and it has wreaked havoc on the ecosystem. There has been a loss of biodiversity in the flora and fauna, as well as a poisoning of the communities that reside in the area. The lack of responsibility taken by both the government and the oil company Chevron (formerly Texaco) has led to many lawsuits, protests, and other forms of organized opposition [38]. Affected communities may benefit from an accessible and sustainable solution to health problems, such as cancer, that have resulted from this unopposed pollution. In this section, we will examine the effects of corrupt oil-government policies on indigenous communities, present the need for collaborative action regarding medical treatment, and explore areas of future research.

As background for the state of contamination in the Ecuadorean Amazon basin, there are a few independent studies that have supplied helpful data. According to an article written by Claudia Garcia [38], the "residents of the Ecuadorean Amazon sued Texaco -acquired by Chevron in 2001- accusing the company of dumping around 80,000 tons of oil and toxic residues on their land between 1964 and 1990 during operations in the Lago Agrio region of northeastern Ecuador. The dumping led to significantly increased rates of cancer, miscarriages and other health problems among the population close to the area" [38]. According to lawyer and activist Pablo Fajardo, even petro-carbon chemical tests completed and unlawfully manipulated by Chevron could not hide the excessively high levels of contamination in the soil and water. Despite these findings, there was little to no action to eradicate this contamination from the area. The potential for economic gain overshadowed the health of current and future populations in the area. This preference of money over human health is completely unsustainable and continues to be supported by industries such as oil.

The process of oil extraction involves many toxic by-products that result in negative effects on human health and the environment. The by-products and residues are put forth into the surrounding air, soil, and water and affect every living thing that makes contact with them. Crude itself also contains many toxic chemicals as crude oil is a complex mixture of many compounds, mostly hydrocarbons. The petroleum hydrocarbons of most toxicological interest are volatile organic compounds (benzene, xylene, and toluene). Benzene is a well-known cause of leukemia and perhaps other hematological neoplasms and disorders [39]. When crude stays in the ground as a true fossil fuel, these harsh compounds are subdued under the earth's crust. When extracted however, they are highly damaging to the environment and living things exposed to it. Yet, we keep drilling for this "liquid gold." This exemplifies the blatant disregard of many operations for medical research that proves negative effects, all for the pursuit of profit.

In a study titled *Exposures and cancer incidence near oil fields in the Amazon basin of Ecuador* by Sebastián et al. [39], the town of San Carlos in northeastern Ecuador is used as a case study for the effects of exposure to these chemicals. In San Carlos, there is almost constant exposure to crude or oil by-products. The oil companies have dumped leftover oil onto the roads, claiming it helps with rising dust (in an area with an average yearly rainfall of 40 in.). Oily roads combined with the 30 oil wells that surround the town and water supplies lead to inevitable daily exposure to crude chemicals. In addition to this, the oil wells surrounding the town have not practiced safe disposal of excess chemicals and instead dumped them into tributary rivers leading to the Napo River. The Huamayalu, Basura, Iniap, and Parker rivers also all run through the village of San Carlos. The town uses the water from the rivers for cooking, washing, bathing, etc. According to the map used in the case study, there are 25 oil wells, 11 within the town boarders, and an oil pumping station directly outside the town's perimeter. The residents of the town not only suffer constant exposure to toxic chemicals; they also spread that exposure to downstream communities through each of the rivers that run through it [38].

The people of San Carlos have endured this exposure for more than 20 years and have suffered many consequences from it [38]. Samples from the water used by the town showed grossly elevated levels of total petroleum hydrocarbons (TPHs) to range from 0.097 to 2.883 parts per million (ppm). For reference, the permitted limit for TPHs in drinking water according to European laws is 0.01 ppm. An article published through Amazon Watch titled *Chevron's Chernobyl in the Amazon* states that "unlike BP's Gulf spill (which received immediate legal action and clean-up efforts) that was a result of a single cataclysmic event, Texaco's oil extraction system in Ecuador was designed, built and operated on the cheap using substandard equipment from the outset [38]. This led to systematic pollution from multiple sources on a daily basis for almost three decades" [39], and yet, Chevron has still succeeded in avoiding responsibility for the damage.

Statistics collected by the San Carlos study showed increased incidences of cancers including stomach, liver, melanoma, leukemia, and more [38]. However, it seems that no one would commit to attributing these elevated rates of cancer to oil contamination. Despite the excess of cancer found in San Carlos and the high exposure to oil pollutants, the attribution of causality to this association has not been forthcoming [39]. Due to the profitability of the oil reserves, these cancer rates among many other ill-health effects seem to have been dismissed. This points to a serious need for action for the health of the people and the environment.

In looking at the *Summary of Independent Health Evaluations of Area of Ecuador's Rainforest Where Chevron Operated from 1964 to 1990* [39], there were three different studies that offered data for significantly increased cancer rates and risks in areas affected by oil pollution. As previously referenced, the piece titled *Chevron's Chernobyl in the Amazon* states that "the court-appointed independent expert in the ongoing trial estimated that Chevron is responsible for at least 1400 excess cancer deaths" [40]. However, these results were denied by Chevron, and the method of diagnosis and data collection was said to have little validity. Chevron also attempted to hide its alarmingly high petrochemical levels of by stating that they were below the US limit. As it turns out, they were just below the US limit for industrial waste water, not drinking water.

According to a study done by Harlee Strauss [41], "no cancer registry was available for the Amazon region and the closest place for diagnosis and treatment was Quito, a 12 h bus ride away" [41]. This made it difficult to place blame on a particular party. Due to the refusal of Chevron to take responsibility and the inaccessible treatment options, it seems that the next step is to offer accessible treatment to the people affected by the contamination. Screening programs to detect health-related problems earlier with appropriate referrals, similar to opportunistic screening clinics organized in other low-resource settings, have the potential to greatly improve health in the area [10] .

Focus on Africa: The Challenge of Defining the Problem in Rwanda: Is Indoor Air Pollution a Health Hazard?

Rwanda is a landlocked republic in Equatorial Africa. The capital Kigali is a typical African city with rapidly increasing development, urbanization, and motorization yet still high rates of open fireplaces and cooking indoors with wood, leaves, dung, and kerosene even in the capital city. Burning wood and other substances for domestic energy is a large source of indoor and outdoor pollution in Rwanda [42]. Suspended particulate matter has been measured and ranges daily from 175 ug/m^3 to as high as 2400 ug/m^3 [43]. For reference, the World Health Organization (WHO) recommended the value for short-term particulate matter exposure is 50 ug/m^3 or less [44]. The meteorological conditions in Kigali further contribute to this health risk by creating increased stability of the urban atmosphere due to the presence of urban heat islands. This results in a lower transportation and dispersion of the polluted air, hence causing accumulation of the airborne pollutants within the small valleys and the residential areas, respectively [43].

To understand how this increase in urbanization and air pollution may be affecting health in general and cancer incidence in particular, we generally turn to cancer registries; however there is no national tumor registry in Rwanda. A literature review of the burden of COPD in Africa revealed that of 22 articles relating to COPD in Africa, only 6 had spirometric data [45]. Only a small number of respondents answered the investigator's surveys despite evidence that they had been received further complicating the difficulty of data collection in a vast continent with communication challenges and limited resources. Indeed, the Global Burden of Cancer [46] used cancer registries, verbal autopsy studies, and other sources to report their findings. Tracheal, bronchus, and lung cancer was the leading cause of death in men and women. At the global level, incidence for women has risen slowly, whereas rates have fallen for men since the mid-1990s suggesting a domestic source of pollution rather than tobacco as the culprit. Lung cancer was the most common cause of death in absolute cases globally as well as in developing and developed regions, yet in Rwanda lung cancer incidence is reportedly <1% [46]. This low rate is highly suspect given that bronchoscopy and pathology services are very limited, there is 1 CT scanner for a country of 12 million, cardiothoracic surgery is unavailable in Rwanda, and chemotherapy is only offered to curable cancers [47]. Lung cancer is not curable without surgery; therefore most cases go undiagnosed, and true incidence is essentially unknown.

Indoor Smoke/Secondhand Smoke Exposure

If cancer rates from indoor air pollution cannot be determined, the next step would be to try to define the incidence of pulmonary diseases. Disease attributable to the environment can be expressed in deaths and in disability-adjusted life years

(DALYs). The latter measure combines the burden due to death and disability in a single index. Using such an index permits the comparison of the burden due to various environmental risk factors with other risk factors or diseases. The realization of how much disease and ill health can be attributed to modifiable environmental risks can contribute to identifying opportunities for prevention and should add impetus to global efforts to encourage sound preventive measures through available policies, strategies, interventions, technologies, and knowledge.

The national burden of disease due to indoor air pollution from solid fuel use was first assessed by the WHO in 2002 [48]. In addition to total deaths and disability-adjusted life years (DALYs) due to indoor air pollution, country-by-country estimates are also available for deaths due to acute lower respiratory infections (ALRI) among children as well as chronic obstructive pulmonary disease (COPD) and lung cancer among adults. Rwanda is among the 20 worst-affected countries [49]. More than 95% of households are exposed to indoor air pollution with 46 DALYs/1000 cap/yr. Total environmental burden of disease per year is 183 DALYs/1000 cap (world range lowest 13, highest 183) with 31% of deaths attributed to environmental risk factors and therefore preventable through healthier environments. Lung cancer rates in 2004 were reportedly low, but tumor registries still are very limited, and in 2004 there were little to no diagnostic capabilities.

Tracheal, bronchus, and lung cancers for men in regions with low smoking prevalence like sub-Saharan Africa are 5–10 times lower than in countries with historically high smoking prevalence like high-income North America, Europe, and East Asia [46]. Despite low smoking rates in Rwanda, lung disease is still highly prevalent, and lung cancer, as outlined above, is likely underdiagnosed. Genetic susceptibility may play a role, but preventable risk factors like household air pollution have also been identified as significant risk factors for lung cancer. According to the latest WHO data published in 2017, lung disease deaths in Rwanda reached 1157 or 1.87% of total deaths. The age-adjusted death rate is 25.79 per 100,000 of populations ranking Rwanda #68 in the world [50].

Awareness is rising, and Rwanda recently joined the International Climate and Clean Air Coalition announcing next steps to reduce pollutants [51]. Although Rwanda does not have many industries, old vehicles, diesel-powered generations, and biomass burning are major sources of pollution in the urban centers. To help reduce pollutants, the government recently increased taxes on old vehicles and introduced mandatory emission testing while urging Rwandans to use cooking gas in the home instead of biomass burning [51].

Conclusion

As the global burden of cancer rises and the cost of treatment approaches unaffordable for many regions of the world, the attention must start turning to prevention.

Vulnerable populations around the world are more susceptible to the harmful effects of pollution, and policies to improve the cleanliness of our air, water, and soil would be a well-spent investment.

The BreatheLife campaign (www.breathelife2030.org), a joint campaign led by the World Health Organization (WHO) and United Nations Environment and the Climate and Clean Air Coalition (CCAC), was launched in October 2016 to mobilize cities and individuals to protect our health and planet from the effects of air pollution and to bring together key messages in a flagship effort to put air quality on the top of health and development agendas. The campaign is not the *only* mode of communicating about air pollution – however it is a means of sharpening messages around technical data and finding new "entry points" for the conversation about air pollution in the virtual world of Internet and social media as well as in the mainstream press [52].

The key components of the campaign model include:

1. *Global campaign platform* – including an interactive website, social media outreach, and videos.
2. *Local campaign "accelerators"* – more intensive campaigns in particular cities, which generate grassroots actions at athletic events and Ted-talk style lectures that can both be promoted by, and inspire, the global effort. This has a multiplier effect insofar as there is evidence that local and national policymakers are often inspired by successful examples of similar actions in their country or region.
3. *Health and environment sector leadership* – it is critical to sensitizing policymakers and the public to both the health *and* climate impacts of air pollution and giving the campaign its unique focus on a people-centered agenda. Using this linkage, environmental policymakers also learn more about the negative health impacts of air pollution, and health policymakers learn more about the sustainability benefits of mitigation [52].

Currently about 14 countries and 26 city-based regions, 2 of which are in Africa, have joined the network, with outreach continuing every day.

Initial response to the campaign was overwhelming, and so one of the key challenges was to respond to success with further institutionalization of campaign tools and tactics. These included:

- Foundational work on the BreatheLife cities network – so as to provide a unique and valuable service to the cities that join
- Continued improvements in the website experience, reflecting new technical advances in data collection, assessment, and visualization, as developed by the WHO and its partners the Global Platform
- Maintaining a constant social media presence, tied strategically to key events
- Developing effective local partners and strategies for local campaigns in cities where the WHO and its partners are engaged in the Urban Health Initiative
- Future fundraising and engagement in new partnerships, including effective engagement with civil society [52]

References

1. Ferlay J, et al. GLOBOCAN 2012 v 1.0. Cancer incidence and mortality worldwide: IARC Cancer No. 11. International Agency for Research on Cancer (online). http://globocan.iarc.fr; 2013.
2. Sloan FA, Gelgank H. Cancer control opportunities in low and middle-income countries. Washington, DC: National Academies Press; 2007.
3. Kanavos P. The rising burden of cancer in the developing world. Ann Oncol. 2006;17(Suppl 8):viii15–23.
4. Flaskerud JH, Winslow BJ. Conceptualizing vulnerable populations health-related research. Nurs Res. 1998;47(2):69–78. PubMed PMID: 9536190.
5. Smith RA, Andrews KS, Brooks D, Fedewa SA, Manassaram-Baptiste D, Saslow D, Brawley OW, Wender RC. Cancer screening in the United States, 2017: a review of current American Cancer Society guidelines and current issues in cancer screening. CA Cancer J Clin. 2017;67(2):100–21. https://doi.org/10.3322/caac.21392. PubMed PMID: 28170086.
6. Waisel DB. Vulnerable populations in healthcare. Curr Opin Anaesthesiol 2013;26(2):186–192. Epub 2013/02/07. https://doi.org/10.1097/ACO.0b013e32835e8c17. PubMed PMID: 23385323.
7. Meneses K, Landier W, Dionne-Odom JN. Vulnerable population challenges in the transformation of cancer care. Semin Oncol Nurs 2016;32(2):144–153. Epub 2016/05/04. https://doi.org/10.1016/j.soncn.2016.02.008. PubMed PMID: 27137471.
8. Atkinson A, Studwell C, Bejarano S, Castellon AMZ, Espinal JAP, Deharvengt S, LaRochelle EPM, Kennedy LS, Tsongalis GJ. Rural distribution of human papilloma virus in low- and middle-income countries. Exp Mol Pathol 2018;104(2):146–150. Epub 2018/03/20. https://doi.org/10.1016/j.yexmp.2018.03.001. PubMed PMID: 29551573.
9. Shastri A, Shastri SS. Cancer screening and prevention in low-resource settings. Nat Rev Cancer 2014;14(12):822–829. Epub 2014/10/31. https://doi.org/10.1038/nrc3859. PubMed PMID: 25355377.
10. Kennedy LS, Bejarano SA, Onega TL, Stenquist DS, Chamberlin MD. Opportunistic breast cancer education and screening in rural Honduras. J Glob Oncol. 2016;2(4):174–180. Epub 2016/03/09. https://doi.org/10.1200/JGO.2015.001107. PubMed PMID: 28717699; PMCID: PMC5497619.
11. Fecht D, Fischer P, Fortunato L, Hoek G, de Hoogh K, Marra M, Kruize H, Vienneau D, Beelen R, Hansell A. Associations between air pollution and socioeconomic characteristics, ethnicity and age profile of neighbourhoods in England and the Netherlands. Environ Pollut 2015;198:201–210. https://doi.org/10.1016/j.envpol.2014.12.014. PubMed PMID: 25622242.
12. Gordon SB, Bruce NG, Grigg J, Hibberd PL, Kurmi OP, Lam KB, Mortimer K, Asante KP, Balakrishnan K, Balmes J, Bar-Zeev N, Bates MN, Breysse PN, Buist S, Chen Z, Havens D, Jack D, Jindal S, Kan H, Mehta S, Moschovis P, Naeher L, Patel A, Perez-Padilla R, Pope D, Rylance J, Semple S, Martin WJ. Respiratory risks from household air pollution in low and middle income countries. Lancet Respir Med. 2014;2(10):823–60. https://doi.org/10.1016/s2213-2600(14)70168-7. PubMed PMID: 25193349; PMCID: PMC5068561.
13. Aelion CM, Davis HT, Lawson AB, Cai B, McDermott S. Associations between soil lead concentrations and populations by race/ethnicity and income-to-poverty ratio in urban and rural areas. Environ Geochem Health. 2013;35(1):1–12.https://doi.org/10.1007/s10653-012-9472-0. PubMed PMID: 22752852; PMCID: PMC4655433.
14. Freire C, Amaya E, Fernández MF, González-Galarzo MC, Ramos R, Molina-Molina JM, Arrebola JP, Olea N. Relationship between occupational social class and exposure to organochlorine pesticides during pregnancy. Chemosphere. 2011;83(6):831–8. https://doi.org/10.1016/j.chemosphere.2011.02.076. PubMed PMID: 21435678.
15. Luzardo OP, Boada LD, Carranza C, Ruiz-Suárez N, Henríquez-Hernández LA, Valerón PF, Zumbado M, Camacho M, Arellano JLP. Socioeconomic development as a determinant of the levels of organochlorine pesticides and PCBs in the inhabitants of Western and Central

African countries. Sci Total Environ. 2014;497–498:97–105. https://doi.org/10.1016/j.scitotenv.2014.07.124. PubMed PMID: 25127444.

16. Maxwell NI. Understanding environmental health : how we live in the world. Sudbury: Jones and Bartlett; 2009. ix, p. 378.

17. Shakeel MK, George PS, Jose J, Jose J, Mathew A. Pesticides and breast cancer risk: a comparison between developed and developing countries. Asian Pac J Cancer Prev. 2010;11(1):173–80. Epub 2010/07/03. PubMed PMID: 20593953.

18. Jørs E, Neupane D, London L. Pesticide poisonings in low- and middle-income countries. Environ Health Insights. 2018;12:1178630217750876. https://doi.org/10.1177/1178630217750876. PubMed PMID: PMC5757432.

19. Dinham B, Malik S. Pesticides and human rights. Int J Occup Environ Health 2003;9(1):40–52. Epub 2003/05/17. https://doi.org/10.1179/107735203800328867 PubMed PMID: 12749630.

20. United States. Environmental Protection Agency. Protect Yourself from Pesticides – Guide for Pesticide Handlers (EPA 735-B-93-003). In: Occupational Safety Branch, editor. Washington, D.C.: Office of Prevention, Pesticides, and Toxic Substances (7506C); 1993.

21. Ntow WJ, Gijzen HJ, Kelderman P, Drechsel P. Farmer perceptions and pesticide use practices in vegetable production in Ghana. Pest Manag Sci. 2006;62(4):356–65. https://doi.org/10.1002/ps.1178. PubMed PMID: 16532443.

22. Danquah AO, Ekor AK, Stella AB. Insecticide use pattern on tomatoes produced at Yonso community in the Sekyere West district of Ashanti region, Ghana. Ghana J Agric Sci. 2009;42(1–2):55–63.

23. Quansah R, Bend JR, Abdul-Rahaman A, Armah FA, Luginaah I, Essumang DK, Iddi S, Chevrier J, Cobbina SJ, Nketiah-Amponsah E, Adu-Kumi S, Darko G, Afful S. Associations between pesticide use and respiratory symptoms: a cross-sectional study in Southern Ghana. Environ Res 2016;150:245–254. Epub 2016/06/20. https://doi.org/10.1016/j.envres.2016.06.013. PubMed PMID: 27318967.

24. Ejigu D, Mekonnen Y. Pesticide use on agricultural fields and health problems in various activities. East Afr Med J. 2005;82(8):427–32. PubMed PMID: 16261921.

25. Negatu B, Kromhout H, Mekonnen Y, Vermeulen R. Use of Chemical Pesticides in Ethiopia: a cross-sectional comparative study on Knowledge, Attitude and Practice of farmers and farm workers in three farming systems. Ann Occup Hyg. 2016;60(5):551–66. https://doi.org/10.1093/annhyg/mew004. PubMed PMID: 26847604.

26. Gesesew HA, Woldemichael K, Massa D, Mwanri L. Farmers knowledge, attitudes, practices and health problems associated with pesticide use in rural irrigation villages, Southwest Ethiopia. PloS one. 2016;11(9):e0162527. https://doi.org/10.1371/journal.pone.0162527. PubMed PMID: 27622668; PMCID: PMC5021266.

27. Mekonnen Y, Agonafir T. Pesticide sprayers' knowledge, attitude and practice of pesticide use on agricultural farms of Ethiopia. Occup Med (Oxford, England). 2002;52(6):311–5. Epub 2002/10/04. PubMed PMID: 12361992.

28. Ngowi AV, Maeda DN, Wesseling C, Partanen TJ, Sanga MP, Mbise G. Pesticide-handling practices in agriculture in Tanzania: observational data from 27 coffee and cotton farms. Int J Occup Environ Health 2001;7(4):326–332. Epub 2002/01/11. https://doi.org/10.1179/107735201800339218. PubMed PMID: 11783862.

29. Bassil KL, Vakil C, Sanborn M, Cole DC, Kaur JS, Kerr KJ. Cancer health effects of pesticides: systematic review. Can Fam Physician. 2007;53(10):1704–11. Epub 2007/10/16. PubMed PMID: 17934034; PMCID: PMC2231435.

30. Clapp RW, Jacobs MM, Loechler EL. Environmental and occupational causes of cancer: new evidence 2005–2007. Rev Environ Health. 2008;23(1):1–37. Epub 2008/06/19. PubMed PMID: 18557596; PMCID: PMC2791455.

31. Parron T, Requena M, Hernandez AF, Alarcon R. Environmental exposure to pesticides and cancer risk in multiple human organ systems. Toxicol Lett 2014;230(2):157–165. Epub 2013/11/26. https://doi.org/10.1016/j.toxlet.2013.11.009. PubMed PMID: 24269242.

32. Leffers J, Smith CM, Huffling K, McDermott-Levy R, Sattler B, Alliance of Nurses for Healthy Environments. Environmental health in nursing. Available from: Alliance of Nurses for Healthy Environments https://envirn.org/e-textbook/.

33. World Health Organization & United Nations Environment Programme. Public health impact of pesticides used in agriculture. Geneva: World Health Organization; 1990.
34. Matysiak M, Kruszewski M, Jodlowska-Jedrych B, Kapka-Skrzypczak L. Effect of prenatal exposure to pesticides on Children's health. J Environ Pathol Toxicol Oncol. 2016;35(4):375–86. https://doi.org/10.1615/JEnvironPatholToxicolOncol.2016016379. PubMed PMID: 27992317.
35. Ferreira JD, Couto AC, Pombo-de-Oliveira MS, Koifman S, Brazilian Collaborative Study Group of Infant Acute L. In utero pesticide exposure and leukemia in Brazilian children < 2 years of age. Environ Health Perspect. 2013;121(2):269–275. Epub 2012/10/25. https://doi.org/10.1289/ehp.1103942. PubMed PMID: 23092909; PMCID: PMC3569673.
36. Chen M, Chang C-H, Tao L, Lu C. Residential exposure to pesticide during childhood and childhood cancers: a meta-analysis. Pediatrics. 2015;136(4):719–29. https://doi.org/10.1542/peds.2015-0006. PubMed PMID: 26371195.
37. Greenop KR, Peters S, Bailey HD, Fritschi L, Attia J, Scott RJ, Glass DC, de Klerk NH, Alvaro F, Armstrong BK, Milne E. Exposure to pesticides and the risk of childhood brain tumors. Cancer Causes Control. 2013;24(7):1269–78. https://doi.org/10.1007/s10552-013-0205-1. PubMed PMID: 23558445.
38. Garcia C. A slippery decision: Chevron oil pollution in Ecuador published September 8, 2016 by Deutsche Welle (dw.com) Permalink: https://p.dw.com/p/1GS5b.
39. San Sebastián M, Armstrong B, Córdoba JA, Stephens C. Exposures and cancer incidence near oil fields in the Amazon basin of Ecuador. Occup Env   iron Med. 2001;58(8):517–22.
40. Chevron's Chernobyl in the Amazon amazonwatch.org ©2000–2018.
41. Expert opinion of Harlee S. Strauss, Phd regarding Human health-related aspects of the environmental contamination from Texpet's E&P activities in the former Napo concession area Oriente region, Ecuador. In the Matter of an Arbitration under the Rules of the United Nations Commission on International Trade Law. Chevron Corporation and Texaco Petroleum Company vs. the Republic of Ecuador, PCA Case No. 2009–23 www.cancilleria.gob.ec February 18, 2013 Prepared for Winston & Strawn, LLP 1700 K Street N.W. Washington DC 20006–3817 and The Louis Berger Group, Inc. 412 Mount Kemble Avenue Morristown, NJ 07962–1946 Prepared by H. Strauss Associates, Inc. 30 Union Avenue Boston, MA02130.
42. Han X, Naeher LP. A review of traffic-related air pollution exposure assessment studies in the developing world. Environ Int. 2006;32(1):106–20.
43. Henninger S. Urban Climate and Air Pollution in Kigali, Rwanda. The seventh international Conference on Urbanization, July 2009, Yokohama, Japan.
44. WHO (2006). Air quality guidelines for particulate matter, ozone, nitrogen dioxide and sulfur dioxide – Global update 2005 – Summary of risk assessment, Geneva, 22 p.
45. Mehrotra A, Oluwole A, Gordon SB. The burden of COPD in Africa: a literature review and prospective survey of the availability of spirometry for COPD diagnosis in Africa. Trop Med Int Health. 2009;14(8):840–8.
46. The Global Burden of Cancer 2013, Global Burden of Disease Cancer Collaboration, JAMA Oncol, 2015;1(4):505–27.
47. Farmer P, Kim JY, Kleinman A, Basilico M. Reimagining global health: an introduction. 2013. University of California Press. Global Health Priorities for the Early Twenty-First Century, chapter 11, p. 323–329.
48. WHO Public Health and the Environment Geneva 2009.
49. www.who.int/quanitifying_ehimpacts/national/countryprofile/rwanda.pdf.
50. worldlifeexpectancy.com.
51. The New Times, Dec 2016.
52. Fletcher E. WHO Communications and Web interface of the Global Platform on Air Pollution and Health. 3rd Meeting of the Global Platform on Air Quality and Health, Madrid, 7–9 March 2017-Meeting Report. p. 51–5.

Chapter 4
Causes, Consequences, and Control of High Cancer Drug Prices

Bishal Gyawali

Cancer is a disease that brings medicine, law, social science, and political science together. When cancer affects a person, it not only affects an isolated individual but also affects the family and social setting in which they operate. Cancer outcomes are obviously related to the diagnosis and available therapy, but they are also associated with the socioeconomic status as well as the politico-legal framework that dictates availability and accessibility to cancer treatment. For example, it is no use having treatments that arise from decades of scientific progress against cancer when the social system is designed in a way that some patients cannot access or afford those treatments. It is meaningless to boast of big separation in survival curves when in reality patients' prognoses are determined by where they live or how good their insurance is [1–5]. Increased risk of death due to inability to afford cancer drugs is a real threat to patients with cancer in the modern era [6]. The cost of cancer care has skyrocketed with the increase in cancer drug costs being an important contributor [7, 8]. In this chapter, I will discuss the rationale behind the high price of cancer drugs, the value offered by these drugs, the sustainability of such pricing, and policies that seek to better link cancer drug value and prices.

Cancer Drug Prices

Cancer care costs include not only the cancer drugs but also the costs of various services, such as the inpatient hospital stays, surgery and radiotherapy services, emergency room visits, and outpatient or provider visits, among others. Currently,

B. Gyawali (✉)
Program on Regulation, Therapeutics and Law (PORTAL), Division of
Pharmacoepidemiology and Pharmacoeconomics, Department of Medicine,
Brigham and Women's Hospital, Harvard Medical School, Boston, MA, USA
e-mail: bgyawali@bwh.harvard.edu

© Springer Nature Switzerland AG 2019   39
E. H. Bernicker (ed.), *Cancer and Society*,
https://doi.org/10.1007/978-3-030-05855-5_4

cancer drug costs account for approximately 20% of the total cancer care costs [7]. So while cancer drug prices are an important part of any discussion of rising cancer care costs, they are not the whole story. Although controlling drug costs doesn't mean other aspects of cancer care costs shouldn't be scrutinized, cancer drug prices are growing at a rate far exceeding the rate of inflation, and cancer drug costs are out of proportion with the value they provide. Finally, it is important to remember that allocating resources for expensive but low-value cancer drugs could mean stripping resources to other high-value interventions [9].

Prescription drugs appropriately draw attention in any discussion of curbing cancer care costs because their prices are increasing at an alarming rate. Growth in cancer drug prices is expected to exceed the growth in total cancer spending [10]. Globally, annual spending on cancer drug costs is expected to increase from $107 billion in 2015 to $150 billion in 2020 [11, 12]. Mean monthly cancer drug costs in the USA increased by more than 500% from less than $1900 in 2000 to more than $11,300 in 2014, after adjusting for inflation [13]. These trends are not restricted to the newer agents—even the costs of some older drugs have continued to rise faster than other health-care costs [14].

The price of a good depends in large part on the purchasing capacity of the consumer. In the past years, cancer drugs were considered expensive and unaffordable only for low- and middle-income countries (LMICs), but more recently, cancer drug prices are too expensive even for high-income countries (HICs). This doesn't mean however that the prices are uniform globally; in fact, they differ widely and cost less in LMICs versus HICs, and there is a big variation in drug prices even within HICs [15]. However, when adjusted for the wealth or the purchasing capacity of the nations, cancer drugs are the least affordable in LMICs.

In 2015, cancer drug spending represented 9.2% of total US drug spending—the highest of any specialty [16]. In 2012, of the 13 newly approved cancer drugs, 12 were priced above $100,000. In 2018, brand-name cancer drug prices have increased, and the newer agents routinely cost more than $12,000 a month. Furthermore, a lot of these drugs are now used in combination, further increasing costs. The combination of nivolumab and ipilimumab exceeded the median cost of a house in the USA in 2016 ($252,000 v $240,000) [17]. In 2017, the first chimeric antigen receptor (CAR)-T-cell therapy approved by the US Food and Drug Administration (FDA) came with a onetime cost of $475, 000 per patient [18].

Drug prices continue to grow higher than inflation after launch despite these high initial prices. Bennette et al. conducted an analysis of pricing patterns after the market launch of oral medications approved by FDA between 2000 and 2012 and found that a 30-day cost for these drugs increased 5.2% on average per year during 2007–2013 (95% confidence interval, CI 3.8–6.5) after adjustment for inflation [19]. These rises in cancer drug prices at and after launch do not correlate with rise in other products or average consumer income. As shown in Fig. 4.1, while the median household incomes have stagnated in the USA, cancer drug prices have soared over the years [10].

Cancer drug prices are not set based on a scientific framework and are not aligned with their clinical value or their innovativeness. One study using the DrugAbacus

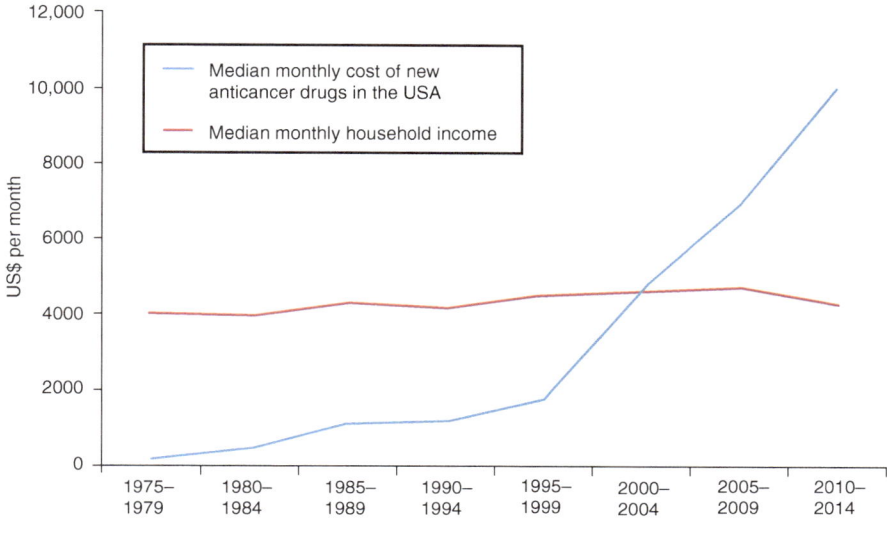

Fig. 4.1 Median monthly cost of anticancer drugs has now exceeded the median monthly household income in the USA and is continuing to rise

tool developed at the Memorial Sloan Kettering Cancer Center showed that almost 80% of cancer drugs in the USA cost more than their value-based price [20]. Such a disproportion has been deemed unsustainable even in high-income countries [21].

High cost of cancer treatment is increasingly being borne by patients. In 2014, out-of-pocket cancer care costs reached $4 billion in the USA [8]. When cancer drug costs impact the real lives of patients, they are no longer just political, legal, or economic issues for academic discussion. Notably, oncologists have been vocal about increasing cancer drug prices. Leukemia experts [22] and other sub-specialists [23] have tried to tackle the cost of new cancer drugs with public appeals to bring the costs down.

Explanations for High Cancer Drug Prices

A frequent argument put forth in the support of high drug costs is the cost of cancer drug development. However, this argument doesn't hold true in economics because what we pay depends more on the value we expect from the product than the cost required in making the product. For example, the cost of a car or an airplane ticket or a hamburger is based primarily on consumers' willingness to pay for the benefit they receive, which is strongly influenced by market competition for alternatives.

Of course, the cost of drug R&D is high. But how high is a matter of debate. A group of economists supported by the pharmaceutical industry used confidential data to estimate the cost of developing a cancer drug at $2.7 billion (adjusted for 2017 US dollars), although that number includes a high cost of capital [24]. Prasad and Mailankody recently conducted an analysis which revealed that the median cost of developing a single cancer drug could be as low as $648.0 million (range 157.3 million–1950.8 million) [24]. The same analysis showed that the median revenue post-approval was $1658.4 million (range $204.1 million–$22275.0 million) [24, 25]. In a median 4.0 (range 0.8–8.8 years) years after approval, 90% drugs had total revenues higher than the R&D spending, and 40% drugs had revenues more than tenfold higher than R&D spending. R&D spending may be much lower for new cancer drugs that are not innovative or novel drugs but are rather next-in-class or me-too drugs. These me-too drugs have lower risk of failure than for the first-in-class drugs; however they often cost as much or even higher than the first novel drug in the class after they are approved. The same authors looked at all cancer drugs approved by the FDA between January 2009 and December 2013 and found that drug prices had no correlation with novelty or efficacy [26].

Another argument put forth in support of high drug prices is the relative rarity of certain cancers and hence a narrow patient pool from which to recoup the R&D costs. However, this argument doesn't explain continued increase in drug prices even when the patient pool for drug use increases. For instance, the price of imatinib (Gleevec) continued to climb despite expansion of target population to include gastrointestinal stromal tumors beyond its initial approval for chronic myeloid leukemia and availability of other competing agents [27]. PD-1 inhibitors were initially approved for melanoma and cost more than $100,000 for a 1 year of treatment. Later the indications expanded to include lung, urothelial, lymphoma, and MSI-high solid tumors, but the price hasn't decreased. Receipt of a supplemental indication or a recommendation in one of the national compendia in the USA related to a non-FDA-approved ("off-label") use increases the target population. However, in a study of oral cancer drugs, receipt of a supplemental FDA approval increased drug prices by 9.9% and a compendia recommendation by 3.2%, although the latter change was not statistically significant. Drug prices increased by 18.8% (95% confidence interval [CI]: 9.0–29.6) for each additional 1000 eligible patients [19].

An important reason why cancer drug prices are high globally is because cancer drug prices are high in the USA. The USA pays the highest cancer drug prices globally because, unlike other governments, US government payers generally don't have the legal authority to negotiate drug prices with the industry. The FDA does not take cost into account when approving drugs, and the Medicare—the largest purchaser of cancer drugs—is prevented by law from negotiating drug prices. Thus, there is no pressure on the industry to lower prices. In fact, brand-name pharmaceutical manufacturers often employ strategies to stop the prices from decreasing, as will be discussed further below.

The Clinical Benefits and Economic Value of Cancer Drugs

Cancer treatment can generally be either lifesaving or life-prolonging. Curative treatments—such as surgery or radiotherapy—can be lifesaving. Adjuvant drug treatment, which is the administration of cancer drugs after definitive treatment, can be lifesaving in some instances if it reduces the risk of recurrence of fatal cancers. However, most cancer drugs are used when the cancer is no longer curable. In such cases, cancer drugs are used with an intention to prolong, not save, lives. Unfortunately, surveys show that many cancer patients in advanced disease stages are unaware of this difference and spend fortunes in the hopes of cure [28]. As a result, many patients continue to undergo active treatment until the end of life, and new cancer drugs that don't help the patients live even for 6 months (versus 4 months even without the drug) keep getting approved, with a price of around 10,000 US dollars a month [29].

Prolonging lives for patients with cancer is obviously a worthy goal. However, most cancer drugs don't prolong lives or do so only modestly. The median prolongation in overall survival provided by the 71 cancer drugs approved between 2002 and 2014 was 2.1 months [30]. Of the 48 cancer drugs approved for 68 indications by the European Medicines Agency between 2009 and 2013, 24 (35%) indications had an evidence of prolongation of survival at the time of approval, and 3 more went on to show improved survival post-approval [31]. In the USA, the FDA approved 67% of cancer drugs between 2008 and 2012 without evidence of improved survival, and of these drugs, only 14% were later shown to actually improve survival [32]. In another example, among patients with non-small cell lung cancer, the median survival between 2000 and 2011 increased by only 1.5 months despite increase in outpatient spending by 23% [33].

Drugs that do not prolong life may also not improve quality of life. Of the EMA-approved cancer drugs between 2009 and 2013, only 10% (7/68) had an evidence of improvement in quality of life at the time of approval [31]. Assessing quality of life is not mandatory in cancer drug trials, and most drugs don't have data on whether they improve, maintain, or degrade quality of lives [34].

One natural question that can arise is how these drugs could be approved despite not showing any benefit in survival or quality of lives. The answer is that they were approved based on benefits seen in surrogate measures such as response rates or progression-free survival (PFS) that may not be correlated with overall survival [40] or quality of life [34].

Thus, many cancer drugs lack evidence to claim that they make the lives of cancer patients longer or better. However, many will still bear high price tags. Because the cancer drugs differ widely in their benefits and toxicities, it is natural to question if the prices of these drugs correlate with their benefits. Value is defined as benefit per unit cost. So, if a drug is lifesaving, it will likely have value even with a high cost. Patients and payers should expect to pay high prices for top-value drugs, such as cancer cures or those that provide a substantial extension in life. However, in most cases, cancer drug prices are not related to value.

Measuring the value of cancer drugs can be controversial because it requires assigning a financial value to human life. Despite this challenge, a number of professional organizations and expert institutions have developed models to assess value of cancer drugs. For example, the American Society of Clinical Oncology launched a value framework in 2015 (ASCO-VF). The framework provides points based on a drug's efficacy, toxicity, and quality of life profiles to calculate the net health benefit, which is then assessed against the cost to make comparisons with other alternative drugs available in the same setting [35]. The European Society for Medical Oncology (ESMO) has also developed a magnitude of clinical benefit scale (MCBS), which takes the efficacy, toxicity, and quality of life into account, but doesn't consider cost [36]. Del Paggio and colleagues looked at the correlation between cost of cancer drugs and their value as assessed by these frameworks and concluded that the magnitude of clinical benefit and drug cost was *inversely* correlated [37]: the worse the clinical benefit from the drug, the higher the drug cost. Another study reached a conclusion that "costs of novel oncology drugs have increased, while clinical benefits of these medications have not experienced a proportional positive change" [38].

As another example, the National Comprehensive Cancer Network (NCCN) has developed evidence blocks in which it categorizes the cancer drugs on the basis of efficacy, safety, quality of evidence, consistency of evidence, and affordability. A study I helped lead has found that the affordability scores had no relationship with efficacy, safety, or evidence level blocks [39]. Others have found that the average price of drugs was not related to improvements in PFS or overall survival (OS) [26].

The Role of the FDA

The role of drug regulators in most countries is to determine whether a drug's benefits exceed its risks. However, that can be challenging for cancer drugs. Because of the emotional power of cancer, regulators may try to be as flexible as possible in approving cancer drugs that have some potential benefit. As a result, the regulatory authorities end up approving cancer drugs even with dubious benefits. There are many ways that drugs with limited benefits can be approved: approval based on surrogate measures, trials in large numbers of patients showing statistically significant results with limited clinical benefit, using non-inferiority hypothesis trials, testing drugs in combination, and using subgroup analyses.

Often, benefits are dubious because they are based on effects in surrogate measures rather than clinical endpoints. Gains in survival or quality of life are clinical endpoints. However, measuring survival takes time, and there is limited consensus on valid measures of assessing quality of life, particularly as the basis for regulatory approval. As a proxy for survival, various surrogates are used such as PFS (defined as the time from therapy initiation until disease progression or death) or response rate (percentage of patients whose tumor has shrunk under therapy). However, definitions of response and progression can be arbitrary; for example, in many trials, growth in tumor diameter beyond 20% is termed progression, and shrinkage below 30% is response, and anything in between is termed stable disease. The use of these surrogate measures is a reasonable basis for approving a drug if (a) the measures correlate well with OS or (b) benefit in OS is confirmed later. But systematic reviews have showed that surrogate measures often don't correlate well with overall survival in most tumor types [40, 41]. Thus, new cancer drugs provide little value to patients because, to be approved, they need not necessarily make patients live longer or live better. They can simply show that the tumor size decreases or it takes longer time for tumor size to increase.

Poor value drugs can also get regulatory approval by chasing statistical significance with overpowered trials. Erlotinib, which costs over $5000 for a month of treatment, was approved for use in combination with gemcitabine in advanced pancreatic cancer despite showing that it improves survival by only 10 days compared with gemcitabine alone in an RCT [42]. By overpowering a trial, i.e., using large number of patients, it is possible to show marginal gains of a few days or weeks as statistically significant. However, such small gains are clinically meaningless or even harmful (considering the toxicities and cost) to the patients. Necitumumab in lung cancer is another such example. In a trial involving 1093 patients, adding necitumumab to chemotherapy showed a gain in median survival of 1.6 months, leading to FDA approval of the drug (which was later priced at over $11,000 per month) [43]. Thus, any demonstration of statistical significance can lead to billion dollar profits from the cancer drugs [44]. This also explains why some drugs move on to phase 3 trials despite showing negative signals in phase 2 [45].

Another way that low-value drugs might be approved is if they are tested in combination without prior testing them in sequence. For example, nivolumab was shown to improve OS versus everolimus in the second-line treatment of renal cell cancer [46]. Naturally, the next logical step was to test and see if nivolumab improved OS when used as first-line therapy. However, the trial instead tested a combination of nivolumab plus another drug ipilimumab in the first line [47]. This trial showed improved survival, but we don't know whether nivolumab monotherapy—which would be cheaper and less toxic than the nivolumab-ipilimumab combination—would also improve OS in the first line.

A final strategy is using subgroup analyses to prove the superiority of a drug in a particular subset of patients. For example, pertuzumab in addition to trastuzumab and chemotherapy as adjuvant therapy for HER2-positive breast cancer was tested in a phase 3 APHINITY trial, which revealed small gains with adding pertuzumab compared with placebo (3-year disease-free survival rates of 94.1% v 93.2%) [48]. However, somewhat better gains in high-risk subgroup of patients were emphasized (3-year disease-free survival rates of 92.0% v 90.2%) for which the drug received FDA approval. The use of pemetrexed for non-squamous subgroup of non-small cell lung cancer is another case of unadjusted multiple subgroup comparisons being made to demonstrate superior efficacy among non-squamous but not squamous cell lung cancer [49].

Effect of High Cancer Drug Prices on Patients

Increasingly, patients are sharing the brunt of high cancer care costs, even when patients have insurance, due to increases in co-payments and high-deductible health plans. The out-of-pocket (OOP) costs borne by patients with cancer in the USA was $4 billion in 2014 [8]. In an analysis between 2011 and 2014, the average per patient OOP costs in the first year after diagnosis were between $3600 and $5500 depending on the cancer type. The OOP costs were the highest on the month of diagnosis and declined subsequently but never reached the pre-diagnosis level [7]. This usually means that the patient and family have to cut down on other daily living expenses or draw from savings to compensate for the extra health-care expenditures. Sometimes, it can even mean treatment nonadherence, bankruptcy, or personal or familial stress. Such adverse outcomes due to economic impact of cancer treatment on patient and family are now collectively referred to as "financial toxicity" of cancer treatment. Financial toxicity refers to all the downstream detrimental effects on the survival, quality, and daily life activities of patients and their families as a result of excess financial strain caused by the diagnosis of cancer. Cancer drugs are a leading cause of financial toxicity in patients [6].

de Souza and colleagues have developed and validated a tool called the comprehensive score for financial toxicity (COST) to measure objectively the financial toxicity in US cancer patients [50, 51]. COST is an 11-item questionnaire including one financial item, two resource items, and eight affect items. Scores range from 0 to 4 for each item, so total COST score can range from 0 to 44, with lower value indicating greater financial toxicity. A limitation of this tool, however, is that this was developed and validated among US patients covered by insurance. Honda and colleagues are working to evaluate if the same COST tool can be used to assess financial toxicity in Japanese cancer patients where public health insurance system is in place, including a cap on out-of-pocket spending [52]. Some forms of financial toxicities are described below:

Reduced Access to Useful Cancer Drugs This is true specially for patients in LMICs where cancer drugs are most unaffordable, public health insurance system is not in place, and all cost must be borne by the patients out of pocket.

Poor Quality of Life Using data from the 2010 National Health Interview Survey, Fenn et al. examined the relationship between financial toxicity and patient-reported quality of life. Their work shows financial toxicity as the strongest independent predictor of poor quality of life among cancer survivors [53]. In another study, 40% and 33% of lung and colorectal cancer patients, respectively, reported limited financial savings, in absence of any future income, enough to sustain the current standard of living for a maximum of 2 months. Compared with patients who had financial reserves of over 12 months, those with limited financial reserves reported significantly increased pain, greater symptom burden, and poorer quality of life. There was a clear dose-response relationship across all measures of well-being [54].

Poor Adherence   Using administrative claims data in the USA, Streeter et al. studied the factors affecting abandonment of newly prescribed cancer drugs. They showed that the odds of abandonment were more than four times higher for patients enrolled in plans with cost sharing of $500 or more compared with plans with cost sharing of up to $100 [55].

Imatinib can be a definitive cancer cure, but adherence is the key [56]. Unfortunately, the average monthly co-payment for imatinib between 2002 and 2011 was $108. Dusetzina et al. showed that the risk of discontinuing imatinib for patients with higher co-payments was 1.7 times the patients with lower co-payments. The risk of nonadherence was 1.4 times higher [59].

Change in Prescription Drug Use   Zheng et al. have shown that patients with a diagnosis of cancer are at an increased risk of changing prescription drugs use, such as skipping dose, taking less medicine than prescribed, delay in refilling, etc., compared with patients without a diagnosis of cancer [57]. In another study, cancer patients who had financial problems delayed or even abandoned medical care more often than patients without financial problems [58].

Bankruptcy   In a seminal study by Ramsey and colleagues using data from Washington State in US Bankruptcy Court for the period 1995–2009, cancer patients were found 2.65 times more likely to go bankrupt compared with people without cancer [60].

Mortality   Financial toxicity could also lead to increased risk of mortality either directly or via inducing bankruptcy. In an important study by Ramsey et al., US patients who suffer bankruptcy after cancer diagnosis were found to have shorter survival versus those who didn't file for bankruptcy (adjusted hazard ratio for mortality of 1.79, 95% confidence interval 1.64–1.96) [61]. Surprisingly, association of financial toxicity and mortality has been found even in countries with public health insurance system such as Italy where patients don't need to pay for cancer treatments out of pocket. In an analysis by Perrone et al., Italian cancer patients who developed financial toxicity were found to be at increased risk of death (hazard ratio 1.20, 95% confidence interval 1.05–1.37) [62].

Controlling the Cost of Cancer Drugs

Some argue that no cost control measures should be exercised for cancer drugs because that would stifle innovation [63]. However, as already discussed, cancer drug prices are not associated with R&D expenses or the novelty of drugs. Perhaps more importantly, because non-innovative drugs that offer little clinical advantages can be approved and priced at whatever the market will bear (even higher than the novel compound at times), the incentive to invest in drugs that have a more substantial clinical impact is reduced. In 2016, there were 803 registered clinical trials testing 20 drugs of the same class (PD-1 inhibitors), in various stages of completion, enrolling

166,736 patients [64]. This enormous redundancy, however, may succeed in getting drugs approved, but does not lead to competition in cost. In fact, PD-1 inhibitors represent one of the highest-priced drugs in cancer. Therefore, an oncology market in which marginal gains in survival lead to drug approval has already stifled innovation.

Another unlikely scenario for cancer drug prices is that the free market economic principles will control prices on its own, because the rules of the free market don't hold for cancer drugs. In a free market, competition drives lower prices. However, cancer drug market defies these rules because cancer drugs aren't commodities of luxury—but of life and death—and because laws and rules at the federal and state level often require insurance coverage of cancer drugs. A patient diagnosed with cancer will not seek out the best value drug but will likely defer to the recommendations of the oncologist, who often has no knowledge of the cost of drugs. Many patients with cancer will try and exhaust all available options rather than chose one with the best value. Because cancer drugs aren't like any other commodities, the current pricing of cancer drugs is unscientific, irrational, and arguably unethical.

Options for controlling cancer drug costs include:

Negotiating Drug Prices

Paradoxically, unlike many other developed countries, US government—the biggest buyer of cancer drugs—is not allowed to negotiate drug prices either through its Part B (inpatient) or Part D (outpatient) drug benefits. The FDA is also only authorized to make approval decisions based on the evidence and cannot consider the issue of cost. No wonder then that the USA pays the highest of most cancer drugs in the world. However, the US government, being the biggest buyer of cancer drugs, has the biggest power to bring down the cost of cancer drugs globally if it engaged more actively in negotiating prices with the industry [65].

One model to negotiate drug prices is value-based pricing or using cost-effectiveness analysis to determine an appropriate ceiling of cost to pay for the given margin of benefit expected with the drug. A value-based pricing strategy would help contain costs by allocating expense to the drugs that benefit the most. As noted in a perspective: "With value-based pricing, all anticancer agents that show a statistically significant difference in a recognized outcome (such as survival) could be approved, but the market price of these drugs would be required to fall within an upper limit in relation to their cost per life-year or quality adjusted life-year" [66]. One problem with cost-effectiveness analysis is that a drug can look cost-effective if the comparator is already priced very high [67], or, in other words, a BMW can look like a bargain when the only other car on the lot is a Ferrari [68]. Cost-effectiveness analyses are also somewhat subjective, and reviews have shown that analyses done by industry-funded authors are more likely to show a drug as being cost-effective [69].

Another model proposed is indication-specific payment, in which the same drug will be priced differently for different indications [70]. Alternatively, episode-based payment or bundled payment models combine the collective costs of care for a patient with a specified condition, over a defined period of time, into a single payment [71].

A good example of price negotiation in action comes from Japan. Having realized that the cost of nivolumab was unsustainable to the country's economy, Japan's health ministry successfully negotiated a whopping 50% cut in the price of the drug and set the price of incoming new PD-1 inhibitor pembrolizumab in the similar range [72]. Japan's government can even negotiate further price cuts on these drugs because the indications have expanded, increasing the eligible patient pool [73]. This also demonstrates that the drugs are originally priced so high that negotiations of up to 50% price cuts are possible.

Another important step that facilitates negotiating by ensuring that poor-quality drugs do not enter the market is using a minimum threshold of benefit benchmark for FDA approval [74]. FDA approval in particular is taken as a benchmark for global efficacy standards. However, when the FDA grants full approval to drugs based on surrogate measures that haven't been validated [75], it diminishes the incentives to produce better quality drugs that improve outcomes and therefore offer value. Furthermore, sometimes the regulatory authorities can be manipulated by the interested parties leading to approval of ineffective drugs [76].

Biosimilars and Generics

Introduction of biosimilars and generic versions of drugs for which the patent has expired can substantially lower drug prices. According to the FDA, the price of generic drugs can reach 80–85% less than the price of brand-name drugs [77]. However, pharmaceutical manufacturers use various strategies to delay the entry of generics [78, 79]. For example, imatinib (Gleevec) was priced at $26,000/year in 2001 which rose to $146,000 in 2016 despite competition in the marketplace. Gleevec patent expired in July 2015, but in a confidential agreement, Novartis paid the generic manufacturer Sun Pharmaceuticals to delay the entry of generic imatinib for 6 months until February 2016. Finally, when generic imatinib was launched, it was priced at about $140,000/year—similar to the price of brand-name Gleevec [80]. On the contrary, LMICs have sometimes exercised compulsory licensing to develop a generic of a drug while it was still on-patent [81].

The price lowering with biosimilars is not as big. The biosimilar filgrastim costs only 15% lower in the USA compared to filgrastim (versus 30% lower in Europe) [82]. Another problem with biosimilars is the low rate of adoption. So, appropriate policy change should be made to encourage a wider adoption of biosimilars and generics whenever available [83].

Reducing Other Wasteful Practices

Other common practices can artificially sustain high cancer drug prices. For example, cancer drugs are commonly sold in large vials, so that a considerable amount of the drug in the last vial is wasted after making weight- or surface area-based dose calculations. Using an online calculator provided by Bach and colleagues, one can estimate the total cost of leftover or wasted drug for top 20 cancer drugs [84]. Reducing such waste could potentially save billions of dollars every year. Bach et al. propose various alternative vial sizes for the drugs and argue that "If all of our suggestions were adopted, it would lower revenue from leftover drug from $1.8bn to $400m and, including the reductions to doctor and hospital mark-ups on leftover drug, would save around $2bn in total. An alternative would be to leave manufacturers free to select their vial sizes but also require them to refund the cost of leftover drug. This could be achieved through certified disposal and a virtual return."

An ineffective way to address this issue, but the one that is now in practice, is to use a fixed dose that uses all quantity of drug in the vial rather than weight-based dose of cancer drugs. Goldstein et al. have shown that just by shifting from weight-based dosing to fixed dose of pembrolizumab in first-line non-small cell lung cancer, an additional $825 million cost would be incurred to the US health-care system in a single year for the additional pembrolizumab that provides no additional clinical value to the patient [85].

Academia or Public Involvement in Clinical Trials

Most of the basic and translational science research that have led to the development of transformative new drugs have come from academia. Federally funded research has a direct role in the innovation of approximately 10–40% of new drugs and a higher fraction of the most important new drugs [86–88]. It seems then illogical to hand over the clinical development phase to industry and allow charging of exorbitant prices for the same drugs that were originally developed using public tax money. Thus, some experts have proposed academic drug discovery, in partnership with the industry, as a potential solution [17]. Although there are a lot of challenges to this approach, some degree of public-industry partnership in clinical trial process itself is feasible. These approaches would challenge the current model in which the risks of failure in early stage of development are entirely born by the public but the profits from later stages of development going entirely to the private sector [89].

Repurposing of Older/Cheaper Drugs

The literature suggests that older, cheaper drugs might be repurposed for cancer treatment [90, 91]. Arsenic for AML, temsirolimus for renal cell cancer, and propranolol for angiosarcoma are some examples of successful repurposing. The ReDO project has a list of evidence for some drugs that could be repurposed in cancer [91]. However, a big obstacle remains the conduct of robust clinical trials to support the use of these drugs, because these drugs, which may have expired patents, will not be attractive to industry. The Anticancer Fund, a not-for-profit organization based in Brussels, works specifically to support the conduct of clinical trials of such repurposed drugs (disclosure: I have previously served as a consultant for this institution). Even when such trials do happen, patients and physicians may be biased against repurposed versus newer drugs [92].

Academia-Led Non-inferiority Studies

Non-inferiority studies have an important role in cancer to discover if lower course, lower dose, or less frequent administration of anticancer agents produce outcomes that are within the range of acceptable risks. For example, the IDEA collaboration showed that a 3-month course of CAPEOX was non-inferior to using a 6-month course of the same as adjuvant chemotherapy for stage III colon cancers, particularly in the low-risk subgroup [93]. Although oxaliplatin is not a particularly expensive by current standards, this shows that collaborative big studies can be done across countries without industry support. Other important examples, particularly related to cost savings include the finding that 3 monthly use of zoledronic acid is non-inferior to monthly administration for preventing skeletal-related events in patients with bone metastasis [94]. Another study showed that a lower dose of abiraterone may produce non-inferior outcomes when taken with food, exploiting food-drug administration [95]. Importantly, whether a shorter course of adjuvant trastuzumab produces non-inferior outcomes to 1 year of the same for early breast cancer has been tested in multiple non-inferiority trials [96]. Many other questions of similar importance such as whether a fixed duration of immunotherapy drugs produces non-inferior outcomes to continuous administration until progression in metastatic setting can be studied using non-inferiority trial design.

Responsible Prescribing

Since spending is driven by prescribing, substantial change can occur at the level of the prescribing physician. Even if individual oncologists don't have the power to bring the cost of cancer drugs down, they can avoid the use of low-value cancer treatments. I have previously summarized a list of certain low-value practices in oncology that can be safely avoided to minimize cost without necessarily compromising efficacy (Table 4.1) [97]. This list is only a guide and should be updated as new low-value practices are recognized. The Choosing Wisely initiative is another example of this sort of encouragement, although it covers only general low-value practices rather than specific details.

Table 4.1 Examples of low-value practices in oncology contributing to financial toxicity

1. Using ramucirumab in the second-line treatment of metastatic colorectal cancer
2. Using anti-EGFR antibodies in the first-line treatment of right-sided metastatic colorectal cancer
3. Using cetuximab for concurrent use with radiotherapy in locally advanced head and neck squamous cell carcinoma
4. Using single-agent ramucirumab for second-line gastric cancer
5. Using G-CSF for the treatment of febrile neutropenia in non-high-risk patients
6. Using chemotherapy toward the end of life
7. Testing CA-125 tests and CT scans for surveillance in ovarian cancer
8. Using sunitinib for the adjuvant treatment of renal cell carcinoma
9. Ignoring cheaper drugs in supportive care
10. Using necitumumab for squamous non-small cell lung cancer
11. Using ramucirumab for non-small cell lung cancer

Adapted from Gyawali [97]

A Note on LMICs

It is not unusual for LMICs to fall into the trap of copy-pasting HICs when it comes to cancer treatment. However, LMICs should set their own priorities and spend only on interventions and drugs that are of high value to them. Although it may be necessary in the short run, it is somewhat paradoxical for LMICs to invest heavily in purchasing bevacizumab for cervical cancer when HPV vaccination and Pap smear tests aren't implemented properly [98]. I refer to this prioritization and implementation of known high-value interventions as the cancer groundshot approach [99]. An important part of cancer groundshot would be to prioritize high-value drugs for the particular LMIC and ensure easy access and affordability to these high-value drugs rather than spend the limited resources on drugs with marginal returns [100]. The economics of cancer drugs in LMICs may vary substantially from high-income countries [89].

Conclusions

Current cancer drug costs are high, not related to R&D costs, and based on what the market will bear in the USA. Such high cost is not only unsustainable in the USA but also leads to real harms to patients by decreasing adherence and increasing bankruptcy as well as mortality. Some reform measures are essential and wouldn't necessarily stifle innovation. However, not doing anything would further stifle innovation by promoting the development of expensive marginal drugs. Several actions are possible to cut down the costs, but there are challenges. But not acting will lead to problematic financial and health consequences in not too distant future.

On May 11, 2018, the US President announced a blueprint to lower drug prices and reduce out-of-pocket costs in a report titled *American Patients First*. This report identifies four key areas of intervention: increased competition, better negotiation, incentives for lower list prices, and lowering out-of-pocket costs. It remains to be seen how these reforms pan out and what impacts they have on cancer drug costs in the USA and globally [101].

Acknowledgments I am grateful to Aaron S. Kesselheim, MD, JD, MPH (Program On Regulation, Therapeutics And Law, Brigham and Women's Hospital, Harvard Medical School), and Saroj Niraula, MD (Cancer Care Manitoba), for important suggestions and edits to the content of this chapter. I am currently a postdoctoral fellow at BWH funded by a grant from the Laura and John Arnold Foundation.

References

1. Ferlay J, Soerjomataram I, Dikshit R, et al. Cancer incidence and mortality worldwide: sources, methods and major patterns in GLOBOCAN 2012. Int J Cancer. 2015;136(5):E359–86.
2. Torre LA, Siegel RL, Ward EM, Jemal A. Global cancer incidence and mortality rates and trends—an update. Cancer Epidemiol Biomarkers Prev. 2016;25(1):16–27.
3. Allemani C, Weir HK, Carreira H, et al. Global surveillance of cancer survival 1995–2009: analysis of individual data for 25 676 887 patients from 279 population-based registries in 67 countries (CONCORD-2). Lancet. 2015;385(9972):977–1010.
4. Boscoe FP, Johnson CJ, Sherman RL, Stinchcomb DG, Lin G, Henry KA. The relationship between area poverty rate and site-specific cancer incidence in the United States. Cancer. 2014;120(14):2191–8.
5. Gatta G, Trama A, Capocaccia R. Variations in cancer survival and patterns of care across Europe: roles of wealth and health-care organization. J Natl Cancer Inst Monogr. 2013;2013(46):79–87.
6. Zafar SY, Peppercorn JM, Schrag D, et al. The financial toxicity of cancer treatment: a pilot study assessing out-of-pocket expenses and the insured cancer patient's experience. Oncologist. 2013;18(4):381–90.
7. A Multi-Year Look at the Cost Burden of Cancer Care – Milliman Research Report. April 11, 2017. Accessed at http://us.milliman.com/uploadedFiles/insight/2017/cost-burden-cancer-care.pdf.
8. The Costs of Cancer. The American Cancer Society Cancer Action Network (ACS CAN). April 11, 2017. Available at https://www.acscan.org/sites/default/files/Costs%20of%20Cancer%20-%20Final%20Web.pdf
9. Health economics: the cancer drugs cost conundrum. Accessed at http://www.cancerresearchuk.org/funding-for-researchers/research-features/2016-08-10-health-economics-the-cancer-drugs-cost-conundrum.
10. Prasad V, De Jesus K, Mailankody S. The high price of anticancer drugs: origins, implications, barriers, solutions. Nat Rev Clin Oncol. 2017;14(6):381–90.
11. The world spent this much on cancer drugs last year. Accessed at https://www.cnbc.com/2016/06/02/the-worlds-2015-cancer-drug-bill-107-billion-dollars.html.
12. Global Oncology Trends 2017: Advances, Complexity and Cost. QuintilesIMS Institute Report. Accessed at https://morningconsult.com/wp-content/uploads/2017/06/QuintilesIMS-Institute-Oncology-Report.pdf
13. Dusetzina SB. Drug pricing trends for orally administered anticancer medications reimbursed by commercial health plans, 2000-2014. JAMA Oncol. 2016;2(7):960–1.
14. Gordon N, Stemmer SM, Greenberg D, Goldstein DA. Trajectories of injectable cancer drug costs after launch in the United States. J Clin Oncol. 2018;36(4):319–25.

15. Goldstein DA, Clark J, Tu Y, et al. A global comparison of the cost of patented cancer drugs in relation to global differences in wealth. Oncotarget. 2017;8(42):71548–55.
16. Mullard A. US drug spending hits $425 billion. Nat Rev Drug Discov. 2016;15:299.
17. Workman P, Draetta GF, Schellens JHM, Bernards R. How much longer will we put up with $100,000 cancer drugs? Cell. 2017;168(4):579–83.
18. Prasad V. Tisagenlecleucel — the first approved CAR-T-cell therapy: implications for payers and policy makers. Nat Rev Clin Oncol. 2017;15:11.
19. Bennette CS, Richards C, Sullivan SD, Ramsey SD. Steady increase in prices for oral anticancer drugs after market launch suggests a lack of competitive pressure. Health Aff (Millwood). 2016;35(5):805–12.
20. Dolgin E. Bringing down the cost of cancer treatment. Nature. 2018;555(7695):S26–s29.
21. Researchers call high cost of cancer drugs 'unsustainable'. Accessed at https://www.beckershospitalreview.com/supply-chain/researchers-call-high-cost-of-cancer-drugs-unsustainable.html.
22. The price of drugs for chronic myeloid leukemia (CML) is a reflection of the unsustainable prices of cancer drugs: from the perspective of a large group of CML experts. Blood. 2013;121(22):4439–42.
23. Tefferi A, Kantarjian H, Rajkumar SV, et al. In support of a patient-driven initiative and petition to lower the high price of cancer drugs. Mayo Clin Proc. 2015;90(8):996–1000.
24. Prasad V, Mailankody S. Research and development spending to bring a single cancer drug to market and revenues after approval. JAMA Intern Med. 2017;177(11):1569–75.
25. DiMasi JA, Grabowski HG, Hansen RW. Innovation in the pharmaceutical industry: new estimates of R&D costs. J Health Econ. 2016;47:20–33. https://doi.org/10.1016/j.jhealeco.2016.01.012.
26. Mailankody S, Prasad V. Five years of cancer drug approvals: innovation, efficacy, and costs. JAMA Oncol. 2015;1(4):539–40.
27. Chen CT, Kesselheim AS. Journey of generic imatinib: a case study in oncology drug pricing. J Oncol Pract. 2017;13(6):352–5.
28. Weeks JC, Catalano PJ, Cronin A, et al. Patients' expectations about effects of chemotherapy for advanced cancer. N Engl J Med. 2012;367(17):1616–25.
29. Gyawali B, Niraula S. Cancer treatment in the last 6 months of life: when inaction can outperform action. Ecancermedicalscience. 2018;12:826.
30. Fojo T, Mailankody S, Lo A. Unintended consequences of expensive cancer therapeutics—the pursuit of marginal indications and a me-too mentality that stifles innovation and creativity: the John Conley lecture. JAMA Otolaryngol Head Neck Surg. 2014;140(12):1225–36.
31. Davis C, Naci H, Gurpinar E, Poplavska E, Pinto A, Aggarwal A. Availability of evidence of benefits on overall survival and quality of life of cancer drugs approved by European Medicines Agency: retrospective cohort study of drug approvals 2009-13. BMJ. 2017;359:j4530.
32. Kim C, Prasad V. Cancer drugs approved on the basis of a surrogate end point and subsequent overall survival: an analysis of 5 years of US Food and Drug Administration Approvals. JAMA Intern Med. 2015;175(12):1992–4.
33. Bradley CJ, Yabroff KR, Mariotto AB, Zeruto C, Tran Q, Warren JL. Antineoplastic treatment of advanced-stage non-small-cell lung cancer: treatment, survival, and spending (2000 to 2011). J Clin Oncol. 2017;35(5):529–35.
34. Hwang TJ, Gyawali B. Association between progression-free survival and patients' quality of life in cancer clinical trials. Int. J. Cancer. 2018. https://doi.org/10.1002/ijc.31957.
35. Schnipper LE, Davidson NE, Wollins DS, et al. Updating the American Society of Clinical Oncology value framework: revisions and reflections in response to comments received. J Clin Oncol. 2016;34(24):2925–34.
36. Cherny NI, Dafni U, Bogaerts J, et al. ESMO-magnitude of clinical benefit scale version 1.1. Ann Oncol. 2017;28(10):2340–66.

37. Del Paggio JC, Sullivan R, Schrag D, et al. Delivery of meaningful cancer care: a retrospective cohort study assessing cost and benefit with the ASCO and ESMO frameworks. Lancet Oncol. 2017;18(7):887–94.
38. Saluja R, Arciero VS, Cheng S, et al. Examining trends in cost and clinical benefit of novel anticancer drugs over time. J Oncol Pract. 0(0):JOP.17.00058.
39. Hwang TJ, Kesselheim AS, Gyawali B. Affordability and price increases of new cancer drugs in clinical guidelines, 2007–2016. JNCI Cancer Spectr. 2018;2(2):pky016.
40. Prasad V, Kim C, Burotto M, Vandross A. The strength of association between surrogate end points and survival in oncology: a systematic review of trial-level meta-analyses. JAMA Intern Med. 2015;175(8):1389–98.
41. Savina M, Gourgou S, Italiano A, et al. Meta-analyses evaluating surrogate endpoints for overall survival in cancer randomized trials: a critical review. Crit Rev Oncol Hematol. 2018;123:21–41.
42. Moore MJ, Goldstein D, Hamm J, et al. Erlotinib plus gemcitabine compared with gemcitabine alone in patients with advanced pancreatic cancer: a phase III trial of the National Cancer Institute of Canada Clinical Trials Group. J Clin Oncol. 2007;25(15):1960–6.
43. Thatcher N, Hirsch FR, Luft AV, et al. Necitumumab plus gemcitabine and cisplatin versus gemcitabine and cisplatin alone as first-line therapy in patients with stage IV squamous non-small-cell lung cancer (SQUIRE): an open-label, randomised, controlled phase 3 trial. Lancet Oncol. 2015;16(7):763–74.
44. Gyawali B, Prasad V. Negative trials in ovarian cancer: is there such a thing as too much optimism? Ecancermedicalscience. 2016;10:ed58.
45. Gyawali B, Addeo A. Negative phase 3 randomized controlled trials: why cancer drugs fail the last barrier? Int J Cancer. 2018;143(8):2079–81.
46. Motzer RJ, Escudier B, McDermott DF, et al. Nivolumab versus Everolimus in advanced renal-cell carcinoma. N Engl J Med. 2015;373(19):1803–13.
47. Motzer RJ, Tannir NM, McDermott DF, et al. Nivolumab plus Ipilimumab versus Sunitinib in advanced renal-cell carcinoma. N Engl J Med. 2018;378(14):1277–90.
48. von Minckwitz G, Procter M, de Azambuja E, et al. Adjuvant Pertuzumab and Trastuzumab in early HER2-positive breast cancer. N Engl J Med. 2017;377(2):122–31.
49. Gyawali B, Prasad V. Pemetrexed in nonsquamous non-small-cell lung cancer: the billion dollar subgroup analysis. JAMA Oncol. 2018;4(1):17–8.
50. de Souza JA, Yap BJ, Hlubocky FJ, et al. The development of a financial toxicity patient-reported outcome in cancer: the COST measure. Cancer. 2014;120(20):3245–53.
51. de Souza JA, Yap BJ, Wroblewski K, et al. Measuring financial toxicity as a clinically relevant patient-reported outcome: the validation of the COmprehensive Score for financial Toxicity (COST). Cancer. 2017;123(3):476–84.
52. Honda K, Gyawali B, Ando M, et al. A prospective survey of comprehensive score for financial toxicity in Japanese cancer patients: report on a pilot study. Ecancermedicalscience. 2018;12:847.
53. Fenn KM, Evans SB, McCorkle R, et al. Impact of financial burden of cancer on survivors' quality of life. J Oncol Pract. 2014;10(5):332–8.
54. Lathan CS, Cronin A, Tucker-Seeley R, Zafar SY, Ayanian JZ, Schrag D. Association of financial strain with symptom burden and quality of life for patients with lung or colorectal cancer. J Clin Oncol. 2016;34(15):1732–40.
55. Streeter SB, Schwartzberg L, Husain N, Johnsrud M. Patient and plan characteristics affecting abandonment of oral oncolytic prescriptions. J Oncol Pract. 2011;7(3S):46s–51s.
56. Darkow T, Henk HJ, Thomas SK, et al. Treatment interruptions and non-adherence with imatinib and associated healthcare costs: a retrospective analysis among managed care patients with chronic myelogenous leukaemia. PharmacoEconomics. 2007;25(6):481–96.
57. Zheng Z, Han X, Guy GP, Davidoff AJ, Li C, Banegas MP, Ekwueme DU, Yabroff KR, Jemal A. Do cancer survivors change their prescription drug use for financial reasons? Findings from

a nationally representative sample in the United States. Cancer. 2017;123:1453–63. https://doi. org/10.1002/cncr.30560.

58. Kent EE, Forsythe LP, Yabroff KR, Weaver KE, Moor JS, Rodriguez JL, Rowland JH. Are survivors who report cancer-related financial problems more likely to forgo or delay medical care? Cancer. 2013;119:3710–7. https://doi.org/10.1002/cncr.28262.

59. Dusetzina SB, Winn AN, Abel GA, Huskamp HA, Keating NL. Cost sharing and adherence to tyrosine kinase inhibitors for patients with chronic myeloid leukemia. J Clin Oncol. 2014;32(4):306–11.

60. Ramsey S, Blough D, Kirchhoff A, et al. Washington State cancer patients found to be at greater risk for bankruptcy than people without a cancer diagnosis. Health Aff (Millwood). 2013;32(6):1143–52.

61. Ramsey SD, Bansal A, Fedorenko CR, et al. Financial insolvency as a risk factor for early mortality among patients with cancer. J Clin Oncol. 2016;34(9):980–6.

62. Perrone F, Jommi C, Di Maio M, et al. The association of financial difficulties with clinical outcomes in cancer patients: secondary analysis of 16 academic prospective clinical trials conducted in Italy†. Ann Oncol. 2016;27(12):2224–9.

63. Easton R. Price controls would stifle innovation in the pharmaceutical industry. First Opinion STAT Accessed at https://www.statnews.com/2018/01/22/price-controls-pharmaceutical-industry/.

64. Brawley L. With 20 agents, 803 trials, and 166,736 patient slots, is pharma investing too heavily in PD-1 drug development? Cancer Lett. 42(37) https://cancerletter.com/articles/20161007_1/.

65. Kesselheim AS, Avorn J, Sarpatwari A. The high cost of prescription drugs in the United States: origins and prospects for reform. JAMA. 2016;316(8):858–71.

66. Ocana A, Amir E, Tannock IF. Toward value-based pricing to boost cancer research and innovation. Cancer Res. 2016;76(11):3127–9.

67. Bach PB. New math on drug cost-effectiveness. N Engl J Med. 2015;373(19):1797–9.

68. Bach PB, Giralt SA, Saltz LB. FDA approval of tisagenlecleucel: promise and complexities of a $475 000 cancer drug. JAMA. 2017;318(19):1861–2.

69. John-Baptiste A, Bell C. Industry sponsored bias in cost effectiveness analyses. BMJ. 2010;341:c5350.

70. Kaltenboeck A, Bach PB. Value-based pricing for drugs: theme and variations. JAMA. 2018;319(21):2165–6.

71. Bach PB, Mirkin JN, Luke JJ. Episode-based payment for cancer care: a proposed pilot for Medicare. Health Aff. 2011;30(3):500–9.

72. Japan sets 50 percent price cut for Bristol Myers' Opdivo cancer drug. Accessed at https:// www.reuters.com/article/us-cancer-japan-opdivo-idUSKBN13C0BD.

73. Japan cuts prices on BMS and Ono's Opdivo, Merck's Keytruda: report. Accessed at https://www. fiercepharma.com/pharma-asia/japan-cuts-prices-ono-s-opdivo-merck-s-keytruda-report

74. Bekelman JE, Joffe S. Three steps toward a more sustainable path for targeted cancer drugs. JAMA. 2018;319(21):2167–8.

75. DeLoughery EP, Prasad V. The US Food and Drug Administration's use of regular approval for cancer drugs based on single-arm studies: implications for subsequent evidence generation. Ann Oncol. 2018;29(3):527–9.

76. Gyawali B, Goldstein DA. The US Food and Drug Administration's approval of adjuvant sunitinib for renal cell cancer: a case of regulatory capture? JAMA Oncol. 2018;4(5):623–4.

77. FDA. Generic Drugs: Questions & Answers. Accessed at https://www.fda.gov/Drugs/ ResourcesForYou/Consumers/QuestionsAnswers/ucm100100.htm.

78. Jones GH, Carrier MA, Silver RT, Kantarjian H. Strategies that delay or prevent the timely availability of affordable generic drugs in the United States. Blood. 2016;127(11):1398–402.

79. Vokinger KN, Kesselheim AS, Avorn J, Sarpatwari A. Strategies that delay market entry of generic drugs. JAMA Intern Med. 2017;177(11):1665–9.

80. Kantarjian H. The arrival of generic imatinib into the U.S. market: an educational event. The ASCO Post. May 25, 2016. The ASCO Post. 2016(May 25, 2016).

81. India orders Bayer to license a patented drug. Accessed at https://www.nytimes.com/2012/03/13/business/global/india-overrules-bayer-allowing-generic-drug.html.
82. As more biosimilars move toward U.S. Market, questions remain about cost savings and uptake by physicians and patients. Accessed at http://www.ascopost.com/issues/november-10-2016/as-more-biosimilars-move-toward-us-market-questions-remain-about-cost-savings-and-uptake-by-physicians-and-patients/.
83. Gyawali B. Biosimilars in oncology: everybody agrees but nobody uses? Recenti Prog Med. 2017;108(4):172–4.
84. Bach PB, Conti RM, Muller RJ, Schnorr GC, Saltz LB. Overspending driven by oversized single dose vials of cancer drugs. BMJ. 2016;352:i788.
85. Goldstein DA, Gordon N, Davidescu M, et al. A phamacoeconomic analysis of personalized dosing vs fixed dosing of pembrolizumab in firstline PD-L1-positive non-small cell lung cancer. J Natl Cancer Inst. 2017;109(11)
86. Stevens AJ, Jensen JJ, Wyller K, Kilgore PC, Chatterjee S, Rohrbaugh ML. The role of public-sector research in the discovery of drugs and vaccines. N Engl J Med. 2011;364(6):535–41.
87. Sampat BN, Lichtenberg FR. What are the respective roles of the public and private sectors in pharmaceutical innovation? Health Aff (Millwood). 2011;30(2):332–9.
88. Kneller R. The importance of new companies for drug discovery: origins of a decade of new drugs. Nat Rev Drug Discov. 2010;9(11):867–82.
89. Gyawali B, Sullivan R. Economics of cancer medicines: for whose benefit? New Bioeth. 2017;23(1):95–104.
90. Bertolini F, Sukhatme VP, Bouche G. Drug repurposing in oncology--patient and health systems opportunities. Nat Rev Clin Oncol. 2015;12(12):732–42.
91. Pantziarka P, Verbaanderd C, Sukhatme V, Capistrano R, Crispino S, Gyawali B, Rooman I, Van Nuffel A, Meheus L, Sukhatme VP and Bouche G. ReDO_DB: the repurposing drugs in oncology database. Ecancermedicalscience. Published online Dec 6, 2018.
92. Gyawali B, Pantziarka P, Crispino S, Bouche G. Does the oncology community have a rejection bias when it comes to repurposed drugs? Ecancermedicalscience. 2018;12:ed76.
93. Grothey A, Sobrero AF, Shields AF, et al. Duration of adjuvant chemotherapy for stage III colon cancer. N Engl J Med. 2018;378(13):1177–88.
94. Himelstein AL, Foster JC, Khatcheressian JL, et al. Effect of longer-interval vs standard dosing of zoledronic acid on skeletal events in patients with bone metastases: a randomized clinical trial. JAMA. 2017;317(1):48–58.
95. Szmulewitz RZ, Peer CJ, Ibraheem A, et al. Prospective international randomized phase II study of low-dose abiraterone with food versus standard dose abiraterone in castration-resistant prostate cancer. J Clin Oncol. 2018; https://doi.org/10.1200/JCO.2017.76.4381.
96. Niraula S, Gyawali B. Optimal duration of adjuvant trastuzumab in treatment of early breast cancer: a meta-analysis of randomized controlled trials. Breast Cancer Res Treat. 2018. https://doi.org/10.1007/s10549-018-4967-8.
97. Gyawali B. Low-value practices in oncology contributing to financial toxicity. Ecancermedicalscience. 2017;11:727.
98. Gyawali B, Iddawela M. Bevacizumab in advanced cervical cancer: issues and challenges for low- and middle-income countries. J Glob Oncol. 2017;3(2):93–7.
99. Gyawali B, Sullivan R, Booth CM. Cancer groundshot: going global before going to the moon. Lancet Oncol. 2018;19(3):288–90.
100. Gyawali B. Cancer drugs in LMICs: cheap but unaffordable. Oncotarget. 2017;8(52):89425–6.
101. American Patients First. Accessed at https://www.hhs.gov/sites/default/files/AmericanPatientsFirst.pdf.

Chapter 5
Clinical Trials: Not for the Poor and the Old

Mary K. Clancy

Introduction

The oncology clinical trial enterprise relies on the voluntary participation of cancer patients. The percentage of adults with cancer enrolled in clinical trials is extremely small and primarily consists of White, insured patients who are less than 65 years of age. Low accrual causes delays and termination of many trials. Skewed study populations result in data that is not generalizable to poor and elderly patients. Inequitable access to oncology clinical trials harms current and future cancer patients. Correcting this inequity is a matter of patient safety and justice. This chapter will review participation rates, factors related to accrual, and potential areas for improvement.

Clinical Trial Participation

Significant disparities have been reported by race and age for NCI Cooperative Group protocols studying breast, prostate, colorectum, and lung cancers [41]. Participants in these trials are primarily White (85.6%) and younger than 65 years of age (68%). Calculations of enrollment fractions (enrollment rates divided by estimated cancer incidence) demonstrate the discrepancies by age and race. Contrast the enrollment fractions for patients aged 65–74 (1.3%) and >75 (0.5%) with that of younger patients (3%) [41]. Elderly patients represent two-thirds of cancer patients, yet they make up only 25–30% of the 2–3% of cancer patients who participate in clinical trials [11, 26, 41].

M. K. Clancy (✉)
Office of Research Protections, Houston Methodist Research Institute, Houston, TX, USA
e-mail: mkclancy@houstonmethodist.org

© Springer Nature Switzerland AG 2019
E. H. Bernicker (ed.), *Cancer and Society*,
https://doi.org/10.1007/978-3-030-05855-5_5

A study of minorities and elderly in multiple myeloma trials [15] provides more evidence that the current clinical trial enrollment system is skewed against the elderly and minority patients. Multiple myeloma is two to three times more prevalent in non-Hispanic Blacks than non-Hispanic Whites, and the average age of diagnosis is 69 years. However, in this study, non-Hispanic Whites were more likely to be enrolled than Blacks (enrollment fraction 0.18% v 0.06%), and elderly patients comprised only one-third of clinical trial participants over a 16-year period, and industry-sponsored studies were less likely to enroll non-Hispanic Blacks than NCI or academic studies (5% v 10%) [15].

Across the United States, poverty is closely related to cancer incidence. Improvements over time seen in other demographic groups for incidence and survival continue to lag for Blacks, due in part to delayed diagnosis, insurance coverage, and less than optimal cancer treatment. The disparity for Blacks is noted across all socioeconomic levels but most notably in underserved communities [46]. Information about socioeconomic status and cancer incidence and mortality enables identification of populations that are "at the greatest risk of cancer diagnosis and mortality and who may therefore benefit from targeted social and medical interventions" [47]. Men and women in the lower socioeconomic groups have 54% and 16% higher mortality rates due to lung cancer and a 30% higher rate of colorectal mortality than those in affluent groups [47].

Federal Guidelines [4] set the threshold for poverty at $25,100 annually for a family of 4 and $12,140 for a person living alone. In 2016, there were an estimated 9.2 million Blacks (22%), 11.1 million Hispanics (21.4%), 1.9 million Asian (10.1%), and 17.3 million Whites (8.8%), with incomes at or below the poverty line. This report included 4.6 million elderly (aged 65 and older) (9.3%) [31]. This does not take into account those individuals and families with significant financial distress due to cancer treatment. Though not officially impoverished, they may be living week to week, on fixed incomes from social security or retirement accounts, and/or employed but underinsured, insured with high out-of-pocket costs, or elderly with no supplemental insurance. In 2016, 4% of adults, aged 18–64, were uninsured. Twenty percent had some form of public insurance [9]. Of privately insured adults, 39.3% with employment-based insurance had high-deductible plans associated with an increased financial burden and delayed care and diagnosis [9]. Many people remain in a "Medicaid gap," "too poor to qualify for subsidies in the new marketplaces, but unable to get into a government program" [7].

Inadequate insurance coverage and patient income are associated with disparities in access to healthcare and, in turn, are associated with lower clinical trial participation rates. It is estimated that patients with annual incomes less than $50,000 are 27% less likely to participate in a clinical trial and that payment concerns in this group are of more importance than randomization when making a decision about participation [50].

Significance

Costs

There are human and financial costs related to inadequate accrual. When trials fail due to lack of enrollment, lagging enrollment, and early participant termination, there are real costs to research sponsors, investigators, and institutions. Estimates of the cost of bringing a new drug from the laboratory through FDA approval vary but may exceed $2 billion and take 10–15 years. This estimate does not include the cost of initiating a study at institutions, the required research infrastructure and staffing at each site [21].

A clinical trial initiated without the reasonable prospect of enrolling sufficient subjects is unethical as it cannot meet the criteria for balanced risk and benefit and its results cannot be relied on beyond the studied population. The patients who do participate may or may not benefit, and their effort is wasted when a trial is closed before completion. Often, the data obtained is not made available to future patients or future investigators. These costs are not calculable.

Generalizability

The inclusion of representative samples in clinical trials is a long-standing problem [11] that affects the reliability of research results and patient safety. FDA guidance recognizes that no research sample will exactly match actual patients and advises physicians to address this problem when interpreting results [21]. In practice, lack of generalizability means that clinicians lack the data needed to interpret results for their patients. The difference between a typical clinical trial population and the "real-world" elderly population seen in a geriatrician's practice is illustrated in Table 5.1 [11]. When the populations vary so widely, it will be difficult to make inferences about the effect of a newly marketed drug.

Table 5.1 Comparison of elderly patients and clinical trial participants

Clinical trial participants	Geriatrician practice
Younger than 75 years of age	80 years of age and older
Minimal comorbidity	Multiple illnesses
Few medications	Multiple medications
Independent daily living activities	Functional decline
Cognitively intact	Cognitive impairment
Able to drive or take public transportation	Limited social support

Created from data in [11]

"The most significant risk factor for the development of cancer is aging" [37]. An estimated 47.8 million (14.9%) US residents are now considered "elderly" (65 years of age or older), and this number is projected to reach 98 million or 25% of the US population by 2060 [10]. Currently, 47% of breast cancer deaths occur in elderly women [25], and it is estimated that deaths in patients 70 years of age and older will soon exceed 50% of all cancer deaths [49].

The rapid aging of the US population and changing racial and minority demographics [15] mean that reliance on data from younger, insured, White patients increasingly fails to provide crucial safety and efficacy data for a majority of the US population. FDA efforts to reduce the timeline to approval for new agents may exacerbate this problem. Drugs approved via the FDA expedited approval program may come to market and are quickly adopted as the standard of care with only "single, nonrandomized, or uncontrolled pivotal trials without patient-relevant outcomes or adequate participation of the elderly and racial or ethnic minorities" [51]. For example, the accelerated approval of immune checkpoint inhibitors (ICI) included limited numbers of elderly in study populations [5].While post-market clinical trials are meant to address these gaps, ongoing ICI therapy is hampered by a dearth of information about dosing, short- and long-term risk, and effectiveness in target populations [51]. In 2016, there were 800 immunotherapy clinical trials requiring an estimated 155,000 enrolled patients [5]. Given the number of clinical trials that fail to enroll sufficient numbers, oncologists may have insufficient prescribing information in the foreseeable future.

Given the potential benefit in clinical trials, and the unknown risks involved in the clinical use of drugs lacking adequate safety and efficacy information, is research any more or actually less risky than clinical care? Is it "really ethical to offer care disengaged from research?" Where does the danger lie when clinicians prescribe treatments whose risks are unknown, without the protections afforded clinical trial participants? [43].

Rights

If access to adequate and equitable healthcare is a civil right, then how should we consider disparities in access to clinical trials and investigational drugs? Patients have a right to information about the risks and benefits of their treatment, and this right is harmed when patients are exposed to risks that are unknown due to inadequate representation in clinical trials. And if clinical trials have the potential of direct benefit, and can be considered as a therapeutic alternative, the rights of patients are protected by appropriately offering the choice of participation; and all efforts need to be made to facilitate access. Oncology practice guidelines reinforce this by stating that patients "should have the choice of participation in a clinical trial at each stage of their treatment…" [52].

The patient advocacy-led Right to Try movement promotes the idea that access to investigational agents is beneficial and, further, is a right; this access "gives life-saving hope back to those who've lost it" [45]. Federal "Right to Try" legislation allows patients to bypass clinical trials after successful completion of Phase I trials and apply directly to a pharmaceutical company for access with no review by the FDA or IRBs despite "almost equally universal criticism from the bioethics, clinical and research communities" [8]. Patients who take this route will receive treatment without true informed consent and the subject protection present in the clinical trial enterprise. This push for greater access to investigational drugs for life-threatening drugs outside of the clinical trial system is a symptom of the problem of low accrual and inequitable access. Too few have access, so a different route has been established.

Equitable access to clinical trials is in keeping with the foundational principles of respect, beneficence, and justice as described by the National Commission for the Protection of Human Subjects of Biomedical and Behavioral Research in the Belmont Report [14]. The interpretation and application of these principles have a direct impact on research participation of the elderly and the poor.

Benefit

Physician attitudes about clinical trial benefit are important as they can act as potential barriers or facilitators to enrollment. In 2002, at a time when enrollment to pediatric trials was at 70%, a study found that 64.1% of pediatric oncologists versus 42.8% of medical oncologists believed that the purpose of a clinical trial was to provide state-of-the-art treatment. This finding contrasted with those who believed that the purpose of a clinical trial was to improve the treatment of future cancer patients [34]. There is concern that the belief that participation offers "state-of-the-art treatment" causes problems for true informed consent since these investigators would be operating under a therapeutic misconception about the purpose of the research [34]. When overestimated, an expectation of benefit for clinical trials contradicts the "raison d'etre of trials, which is to determine whether a drug has value relative to the standard of care"[38]. With the possible exception of first-in-human drugs, there is potential for benefit in most trials.

Modernization of clinical trial design has been accompanied by direct patient benefit that is similar to some FDA-approved drugs. With the use of new immunotherapies, molecularly targeted agents, enrollment of enriched populations more likely to benefit, and designs that look for signals of activity, participation in Phase I trials can result in direct benefit. Patients who participate in Phase I trials "may experience improved quality of life, psychological benefit, and direct medical benefit" [52]. Despite the increased likelihood of direct benefit, ASCO acknowledges the potential for misconception about the purpose of Phase I trials and recommends education for investigators involved in the informed consent process as well as educational videos and material for patients to assure a balanced presentation [52].

There is some evidence of improved outcomes for participants on clinical trials independently of the outcome of the trial or whether they received the investigational or control treatment. This benefit may result in part from the additional oversight and engagement of different members of the research team, follow-up by research coordinators, adherence to protocols, and scheduled clinic visits. A meta-analysis focusing on randomized clinical trials in women's health population found that there was a benefit, better health outcomes for those who participated than for those who received standard care [43].

Institutional Review Boards (IRBs) are required to assess the risks and benefits of a clinical trial prior to approval. By approving a clinical trial, the IRB makes determination that the risks of the research are balanced by the potential benefit, accrued directly by the participant or, indirectly, to future patients (FDA) [19, 20].

Respect and Justice

Respect is shown by acknowledging an individual's autonomy to make decisions in his or her best interest and providing information that is necessary to make that decision in a manner free of coercion and undue influence. Justice requires a fair distribution of risks and benefits and participant selection based not on convenience but justified for scientific reasons. However, respect and justice also require the protection of patients who may lack the capacity for autonomous decisions and those who are vulnerable to coercion or undue influence [14]. The mandates for assurance of autonomy and the protection of the vulnerable often conflict, and if protection becomes paternalism, respect for the individual is lost. Injustice would occur when potentially eligible patients are not asked to participate because of decisions based, unfairly, on group characteristics.

Dorothy Height, a member of the National Commission for the Protection of Human Subjects of Biomedical and Behavioral Research, remembers learning, in contrast to what was expected, that Black prisoners felt unfairly excluded from research because the White prisoners who did participate received additional benefits, including early release. Ironically, Black prisoners were excluded out of concern that they were vulnerable and had been subject to injustice [30]. Decades after the publication of the Belmont Report, Dr. Height would call for renewed attention to the mandate for justice, stating "even if there were no excellent scientific reasons to eliminate the disparities in clinical trials–which there are-the need for justice in human participation research alone justifies the effort."

Contributing Factors

There are many, often cited, factors related to clinical trial participation that apply across all types of trials, cancer diagnoses, and demographic groups. However, we should keep in mind the primary reason that patients don't enroll in a clinical trial.

They are not asked [29, 30, 41].

Cancer patients are not asked to participate in a clinical trial for a multitude of reasons, driven by study design, beliefs and attitudes, regulations, or economics.

Clinicians

What prevents primary care physicians, nonacademic oncologists, and even oncologists and investigators, at premier cancer centers, from taking the basic step of informing a patient of all possible alternatives to care? Since the treating provider makes the decision about offering trial participation to his or her patient [15], understanding and addressing these factors are critical. Factors that may affect physicians' decisions include belief that standard of care is better, or that the treatment in clinical trials is no better, concern about unknown risks, reluctance to rely on randomization for treatment decisions, competing trials, concern about patient compliance and the time and documentation required by the clinician and staff, and concern that their patients will be lost to another practice [15, 23, 29, 39].

Clinicians may simply be out of time. For many oncologists, 49% of clinical time is consumed by electronic health record requirements [3]. To participate as an investigator, oncologists must obtain training in human subject research ethics, FDA Good Clinical Practice, other regulations, and protocol-specific training. As a principal investigator, they will be responsible for study oversight, delegation of duties to a research team, assessment and documentation of eligibility, procedures, adverse events, site initiation meetings, and meetings with monitors and internal auditors as well as financial responsibilites.

Negative attitudes toward research may be a result of the same negative press available to patients and their families. Required training about research ethics, responsible conduct, and regulations related to human subject research begin with historic and current accounts of research scandals and misconduct. Meant as cautionary tales, the scandal of research may be the unintended take-home message. In some cases, that is the intent. Consider a report entitled "The Anatomy of Research Scandals" [16] in which the author discusses a seminar on medical research that he designed to "crush the idealism of future physicians by illuminating the dark patterns that research scandals typically follow."

Eligibility Criteria

Clinical trial eligibility criteria are designed to reduce heterogeneity and risks, known and theoretical, and to increase the likelihood that noted effects are due to the study drug [33] and are driven, as well, by an FDA approval process relying on efficacy and internal reliability, not effectiveness and safety [11]. So, these demands result in eligibility criteria that have increased in number and specificity over time resulting in a cascade of effects that include delayed enrollment, decreased generalizability, and increased complexity and costs [26].

Despite the 1989 FDA Guidance that stated "there is no good basis for the exclusion of patients on the basis of advanced age alone, or because of the presence of any concomitant illness or medication…" [11], age continues to be a limiting factor for clinical trial participation. In 2005, it was reported that "Age is no longer a valid eligibility criterion" and that most studies did not have a specific upper age limit. However, a significant reduction in recruitment of elderly patients with cancer occurred when exclusion criteria included "hypertension, cardiac disease, hematologic, or pulmonary function abnormalities," and mild to moderate reduction in functional status [49]. Concerns about compliance, family influence, transportation, and comprehension can mean that an elderly patient is not asked. The most common reasons cited by physicians who decided against a clinical trial were that the treatment was considered too toxic (33%), the best treatment was not included in the available clinical trials (27%), and the physician was unaware that a trial was available (21%). Medical care of the elderly is complicated by comorbid conditions, multiple medications, isolation, access, and need for support services (FDA), all of which may make a person ineligible or act as a barrier for an otherwise eligible patient. Elderly may also be excluded because they "have a greater likelihood of getting sick or dying during the trial" a not insignificant concern for a study sponsor [11].

The effects of healthcare disparities in the poor that result in higher cancer incidence and mortality [46] are likely to result in decreased access to clinical trials or exclusion. Like the elderly, the poor may be excluded from clinical trials due to comorbidities and past medical history. They are also negatively impacted by delayed access to care and advanced disease at the time of diagnosis. Patients living in areas with inadequate numbers of oncologists per patient are less likely to have access to clinical trials, and those that must travel, due to rural residence or distance from a cancer center, may not be able to participate for studies that require frequent visits. This is not specific to the poor and elderly, but any additional burden will have greater negative effects in these populations.

Cost

Clinical trials do not specifically exclude patients based on socioeconomic status (SES), but SES and insurance status certainly play a de facto role. As genetic markers and other new and expensive testing are used for diagnosis and eligibility, the poor, and poorly insured, will be less likely to be enrolled [15]. And, because most cancer costs occur in the elderly, rising costs will negatively impact their enrollment as well. Elderly cancer patients relying on Medicare alone can have out-of-pocket (OOP) costs as high as 60% of their annual income [42].

According to verywellhealth.com, a patient sites "clinical trials are not free. Someone does have to pay, but for the vast majority of the time, it is not the patient who is paying. A majority of clinical trials are federally or privately funded, so there is no cost to the participant" [18]. While it is true that "clinical trials are not free," patients do pay for participation in clinical trials. Insurance coverage reimburses for routine costs of care associated with clinical trials. However, the determination of which treatments and procedures constitute "routine" or "standard" care differs by institutions, states, and insurers. A favorable outcome for a patient often relies on the best efforts of their oncologist [48].

Research Infrastructure

Successful clinical trial sites require an infrastructure that, in addition to having qualified investigators and research teams, has adequate clinical and administrative personnel and space, specialized equipment, and clinical time and expertise. This includes teams that are capable of conducting accurate feasibility assessments, clinical trial budgets, research billing and regulatory submissions. Inadequate planning and unrealistic feasibility assessments do not adequately address the time and effort required to enroll the agreed-upon number of research patients. Gaps in staffing may result in delayed study start, recruitment, and enrollment. Ongoing recruitment and enrollment are often sacrificed when a research team finds itself short-staffed since the management of current research patients has to be a priority. Failure to address these issues result in studies that close due to lack of enrollment or studies that simply linger on costing the sponsor and site both time and money.

Institutions that provide care for underserved, vulnerable populations may decline site initiation due to the cost of study start-up and lack of clinical research resources and staff ready to perform complex study procedures [27]. Clinical trial finance, including coverage analysis, and financial assistance to potential participants are cited as an area that requires study in order to expand access to "safety net" hospitals.

Coverage analysis is conducted for all clinical trials to determine which costs are assigned to study sponsors (i.e., research components) and which to the patient and/or third-party payers (i.e., standard-of-care components) [27]. The time and effort spent on coverage analysis for each clinical trial is costly and time-consuming and can result in conflict because there is no "standard" for standard of care [48]. A research patient may understand from the consent process that the cost of a procedure is covered by the "research" when the finance team has made a different decision. The cost for this analysis consumes resources that could otherwise be used for patient accrual.

In practice, the difference between cancer research and clinical care is narrow. The FDA exempts oncology trials from IND requirements when the design, population, dosage, or route does not significantly increase the risk of a marketed drug [22]. Oncology is granted this exemption because oncologists, backed by clinical evidence and experience, routinely utilize drugs off-label and try different combinations and regimens for drugs with significant risk of toxicity. Because oncology practice can vary widely, based on physician experience and patient need, it seems that the procedures deemed "research" only in the coverage analysis process would be relatively few.

Patients

When asked to participate in a clinical trial, an eligible cancer patient is presented with a consequential choice requiring complex decision-making at a time of great personal stress. They must process information about the purpose of the research, differences between research and standard approaches, control over treatment, risks and benefit, time and effort, inconvenience, insurance coverage, and other costs [53]. These factors are weighed against the patient's belief system, culture, family, education, experience, and trust. After an initial discussion, the patient may leave with a 30-page informed consent document summarizing the research. It will include pages of risks and a brief sentence or two about the benefits. For example, "Benefit is not guaranteed." "This study is not designed to benefit you." "Future patients will benefit." This multifactorial process is stacked against the risk of participation.

Potential participants are affected by societal attitudes and information from patient-directed marketing and media. Patients arrive having been subjected to conflicting, subliminal, messages concerning the beneficence or maleficence of biomedical research. If a patient reads US News & World Report, they understand that the "best" hospitals conduct clinical trials [13]. Academic medical centers promote the idea that clinical trial participation is beneficial by linking access to clinical trials with access to innovative treatments and procedures [38]. Headlines in mainstream and professional news sources use terms like "miracle," "cure," "groundbreaking," "home run," "revolutionary," and "marvel" [1], and the FDA applies designations such as "breakthrough therapy" to reduce time to approval and make these drugs available as soon as possible [51]. These terms confuse the potential benefit of investigational drugs and the benefit of clinical trials. At the same time, the media promotes a negative perception of clinical research and healthcare generally. Headlines about research misconduct, noncompliance, conflict of interest, and profiteering tend to reduce trust in the system and may influence a patient's decision to participate in a clinical trial.

A survey of primarily White, well-educated, employed patients identified four main attitudes or concerns about participation in a clinical trial. These were fear about side effects, insurance coverage, lack of efficacy, and receipt of a "sugar" pill. College-educated patients and those with metastatic disease or prior clinical trial experience had fewer negative attitudes [39]. There continues to be evidence that past transgressions have not been forgotten by minority groups, specifically in the Black population, [41] but education and income also affect trial participation. Results of a survey of patients in rural North Carolina and patients at the Duke Cancer Clinic found that fewer Black patients than Whites were willing to participate in a clinical trial. However, the greatest difference between the groups was not race but education and income. Lower education, income, and the belief that God would determine outcome were correlated with less willingness to participate [2].

Some patients may arrive at clinic asking to participate in clinical trials due to results of their online searches. These patients may be more likely to enroll on a trial but may also have assumptions that need correction because information is not readily accessible and may not be understandable. Clinicaltrials.gov, with 200 million page views per month [36], is written by sponsors to meet regulatory requirements, not for patients searching for trials, and the reading level is far above the average patient's literacy level.

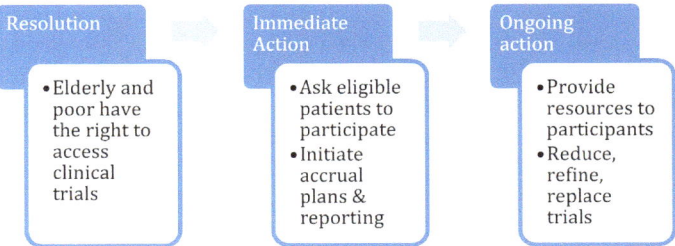

Fig. 5.1 Action plan

(Re)Solutions

Clinical trial disparities have been noted for decades, and despite repeated calls for action and initiatives, the problem is essentially unchanged. At the Federal level, the Cures Act and the Moonshot have stimulated collaboration among federal agencies, industry, and academia that is focused on patient engagement, a coordinated work-force, and equitable access [3]. There is an enthusiasm for change. However, the consensus needed for true change, followed by legislation, guidance, and imple-mentation, will likely take years to accomplish. While federal initiatives progress, there is still much that can be done, starting with each investigator, study coordina-tor, research nurse, social worker, institution, IRB member, sponsor, and funding agency (Fig. 5.1).

Resolution

Minds and hearts are not easily moved from long-held beliefs and attitudes, but this is necessary if there is to be general acceptance of an individual's right to participate in an applicable clinical trial. For this to happen, investigators and members of the research team responsible have to be able to verbalize why access is critical as a matter of justice and beneficence. Otherwise, they will continue to be reluctant to give all eligible patients the opportunity to participate.

A shift in perspective for IRBs is also needed, one that moves from, primarily, a protective stance to a more balanced review process that assures the individual's right to make a voluntary autonomous decision. IRB review must fully incorporate the principle of justice.

Immediate Action

Simply asking eligible patients to participate would significantly increase the rate of enrollment. This should involve an active process that begins before a patient arrives at a cancer center. Patients are often sent links with information and health question-naires that must be completed before their first appointment. An introduction to the center should include information about clinical trials and links to cancer resources and active trials at the site. Basic brochures about the purpose of clinical trials should be available in the waiting rooms. This would provide some awareness of clinical trials before a patient is asked to participate. All members of the research team should be aware of, or have access to, information about applicable clinical trials. A navigator or recruitment coordinator would be responsible for reviewing all patients scheduled for visits and providing relevant information to the clinical and research teams to assure that applicable patients are at least considered for participation.

Protocol feasibility assessments that include accrual factors, not just the number of patients at a given site, would increase the likelihood that a study will enroll not just the required number of participants but also includes a representative sample. A tool that incorporates known barriers [6] would identify trials at high risk for low accrual and could be used to develop realistic accrual plans and timelines. Sponsors and sites can then determine if a trial is worthwhile, even if there is a need for an extended enrollment period or significant resource allocation. These resources may include staff to identify and recruit the elderly and an assessment and provision of patient transportation and home support [49]. Each site would use this plan to assure that enrollment stays on track. Clinical trials accrual plans that specifically address inclusion of the poor and the elderly and include measures that would enable par-ticipation should be required and reviewed by funding and regulatory agencies. An immediate impact would be made if this was fully adopted for NCI Cooperative Group trials [25].

IRBs must review eligibility criteria to assure that the exclusion criteria are fair and are justified by the science (FDA), but review of accrual plans may be viewed as "IRB scope creep." Assuming that enrollment study wide will be equitable, a local IRB, reviewing a multicenter clinical trial, may not take up the issue even though the population at the local site is limited. Increased reliance on central or single IRBs may present an opportunity for change. Central IRBs have the respon-sibility for review of an entire trial. As a matter of justice, CIRBs must review for equitable inclusion and, as a matter of risk, must assess the feasibility of a trial. They can require submission of an accrual plan. Nationally, CIRBs have the means to assure justice for the poor and elderly who have not been included to date.

Ongoing Action

Industry sponsors can address the barrier posed by the cost of cancer care and the incremental cost of trial participation by establishing methods to reimburse for travel expenses. Reimbursement for expenses is a measurable response that reduces barriers to participation while avoiding the concern of undue influence. However, these modest measures may not be sufficient for patients whose financial status represents a barrier to adequate healthcare. Improving access to cancer trials by "erasing the stigma of undue inducement" is the objective of the Lazarex Cancer Foundation, a philanthropic organization that supports access by providing reimbursement to research patients who could not afford the out-of-pocket costs of participation [35]. Lazarex is working to reduce the health access disparity created by current misconception and lack of guidance surrounding reimbursement for the ancillary (incremental) costs of participation and have launched an initiative with the 10-year goal of eliminating this barrier to clinical trial participation. In partnership with the Lazarex, an innovative "cancer care equity program (CCEP)" was established to address the direct costs of participation that act as barriers to participation in clinical trials. Financial assistance was provided for travel, lodging, and other trial-related expenses to patients who passed a financial screen. The program has resulted in increased enrollment for enrollees whose financial status would have prevented clinical trial participation [44]. This is a model that should be adopted by other cancer center foundations and philanthropic organizations.

Institutions could effectively reduce barriers to clinical trial participation by treating all patients the same. Academic medical centers that have a system to provide "charity care" have the opportunity to assist research patients who meet basic financial criteria. Potentially eligible research patients referred from community clinics staffed by AMC residency programs could automatically be referred to appropriate care navigators and the oncology recruitment coordinator.

As a group, very poor cancer patients are considered vulnerable to undue influence (FDA), and it is the IRBs' responsibility to assure that payment or compensation does not take precedence over other important factors such as purpose, procedures, or risks of the study in a patient's decision to participate. IRBs routinely approve some level of compensation. However, payment to research subjects is subject to greater scrutiny despite evidence that payment "obscures the risk perception of potential research participants" [28]. IRBs are cautioned against the mistake of equating poverty with lack of capacity and further restricting an individual's options [28]. Greater compensation for participation may lower the barriers to enrollment for the poor without harm.

Patient burdens related to travel, across town, or from rural areas, could also be reduced through the use of telemedicine [3]. ASCO provides several examples of successful telemedicine programs for small, rural, and large-scale systems that result in increased patient satisfaction, fewer emergency room visits, and minimal increase in physician workload. These programs could be implemented to reduce the number of trips to a cancer center.

Reduce, Refine, and Replace

The principles of reduction, refinement, and replacement have been adopted in arenas where unnecessary and/or inefficient use of subjects or materials results in harm. They are a useful way to think about the current inequity in oncology clinical trials and some potential changes (Fig. 5.2).

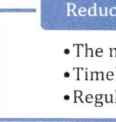

Reduce
- The number of clinical trials
- Timeline for accrual and terminate trials not meeting accrual goals
- Regulatory and financial burdens

Refine
- Study designs and statistical plans to account for the human element
- Informed consent language by providing key elements in initial concise summary
- Coverage analysis for clinical trials

Replace
- Later phase clinical trials with observational data, use of electronic health record and data routinely reported
- Mixed messages about research with accurate, balanced, targeted information
- Passive accrual process with proactive, protocol and site specific plans and action

Fig. 5.2 Resolutions

Reduce

Too many clinical trials are competing for the same patient populations. For example, the annual number of new cases of breast cancer in the United States is estimated at 252,710. In the same time period, 275,342 participants were required for 533 breast cancer trials listed in a clinicaltrials.gov search [12]. Many of these studies will be closed due to low accrual and would never have been opened if an accurate feasibility assessment and accrual planning had been done. The dollars, time, and effort involved in opening and maintaining a low-functioning trial are better used elsewhere. Funding agencies, Data Safety Monitoring Boards, and Investigator sites should track and close trials that fail to meet accrual timelines.

Regulatory burden negatively impacts accrual in several ways. Assuring compliance with research regulations takes time that clinical investigators could better use to review patient histories, have meaningful consent conversations with potential participants, and write or provide feedback about trial designs and eligibility criteria that would facilitate participation by elderly and poor cancer patients.

The current clinical trial consent document includes pages of required language that distract from the core elements. FDA guidance on minimum, or maximum, requirements for the description of risks, for example, would be helpful. Is information about the pain of blood draws really needed? The discomfort of ECG sticky pads? What type of information could be placed in an addendum, or just excluded? Informed consents should have less, better, information. Sites should be encouraged to implement alternative formats such as the electronic consent forms.

Modified regulatory requirements for clinicians who may only be engaged tangentially would allow them to support their patients who are in clinical trials without being added to the research team. This could foster collaboration with oncologists who are reluctant to refer a patient for a clinical trial because they may lose them to their practice. It would enable them to conduct standard clinic visits, perhaps manage their patients in a private office distant from the cancer center but support the research in some way.

There is a chasm between medical practice and clinical research that prevents clinicians and patients from participation. The 1979 Belmont Report made a distinction between medical practice, which is designed "for the well-being of an individual patient," and research, which is designed to "test a hypothesis" and "develop or contribute to generalizable knowledge" [14]. The purpose of each is different but complementary. In the decades following the Report, regulations, guidance, oversight, review processes, and education and training requirements have emphasized the differences between clinical practice and research. Oncology practice routinely involves treatment combinations that are off-label [22]. No additional consent or oversight is needed for this. But when these same combinations are included in a trial designed to obtain objective data, the same clinician faces an entirely different set of rules. Yes, research is "for future patients," but the care that is provided in a clinical trial is about the research patient. Trials include data and safety monitoring that protect current patients, and clinical investigators can stop participation at any time based on the research patient's best interest. Quality improvement initiatives and data collected for reporting purposes are considered to be part of clinical practice or hospital operations. It is possible to reduce the number of clinical trials by utilizing the vast array of clinical data available via electronic health records, registries, and quality reporting and by moving to a learning healthcare system [3, 17].

Refine

Study designs should account for slow accrual, early withdrawals or loss to follow-up, participant burden, and cost. Rigorous randomized clinical trials fail when these elements are not included. Designs that adhere more closely to the standard of care, e.g., pragmatic design or others, might be better positioned to meet accrual goals and study objectives [24]. Designs that provide crossover to treatment arms and continued access may add potential benefit to research patients initially assigned to placebo or who are enrolled in early phase trials.

The informed consent processes for practice and research need to fully inform patients about the known and unknown risks and benefits of treatment options. Greater transparency about the knowledge deficits in drugs prescribed in usual practice would allow patients to make more informed choices when asked to participate in research. Consistent with the anticipated changes to the Common Rule, informed consent documents for all clinical trials should start with a concise summary that in very few words explains that participation is voluntary, the purpose of the research and its risks and benefits [40]. This concise summary could also be used as the standard summary provided for patients in clinical trial websites.

Refinement, guidance, and simplification are needed in the coverage analysis process that determines what procedures will be charged to the research study and which are the responsibilities of the insurer and research patient. Sponsors should accept responsibility for initiating a coverage template for each trial or, at least, identifying those procedures considered "research only." A system where sponsors provide sites with protocol-specific coverage analyses, followed by confirmation at a site, would reduce time to study start-up and also more fairly and uniformly assign benefits study wide. Cost savings could be used to hire social work staff and financial navigators to work with patients to reduce financial barriers to care and to clinical trials.

Replace

Continuous evaluation of safety and efficacy for approved drugs, especially those that are approved with reduced requirements, is needed. However, post-market trials compete with trials of new treatments and combinations that include the same patient populations. Phase IV trials could be replaced via existing reporting mechanisms and rely on real-world reporting instead of enrolling patients in clinical trials. Pragmatic trials, closely aligned to clinical practice [24], observational studies, registries, and use of existing data and electronic health records and administrative and claims databases are all potential sources of long-term safety data [11].

The clinical trial enterprise needs to better "control the message" about the importance and potential benefit of clinical trials. Press releases about advances in science need to include balanced expectations for timelines and potential benefits. Institutions can develop population-specific material about cancer clinical trials for patients at the cancer center and surrounding community outreach clinics [2]. More patient-centric sites are needed to enable searches that meet a patient's specific needs. For example, is there a trial for a patient like me [32, 36]?

Most importantly, the expectation that an eligible research patient will appear when needed and will consent to participation must be abandoned. To assure adequate and equitable enrollment, current passive accrual processes must be replaced with proactive protocols and site-specific plans and action, followed by review and reporting, enabling continuous quality improvement in this area. Patients that reflect the anticipated patient population, the elderly, and the poor must be included in the conversation. Not as research subjects but as true partners.

Clinical trials rely on the voluntary participation of patients with cancer. Future patients rely on data provided by patients like them. Current patients have the right to know all therapeutic options and have access to applicable clinical trials. This all starts with just asking. Ask.

References

1. Abola MV, Prasad V. The use of superlatives in cancer research. JAMA Oncol. 2016;2:139–41. https://doi.org/10.1001/jamaoncol.2015.3931.
2. Advani AS, et al. Barriers to the participation of African-American patients with cancer in clinical trials: a pilot study. Cancer. 2003;97:1499–506.
3. ASCO. The state of cancer care in America, 2017: a report by the American Society of Clinical Oncology. J Oncol Pract. 2017;13:e353–94. https://doi.org/10.1200/jop.2016.020743.
4. ASPE. U.S. Federal Poverty guidelines used to determine financial eligibility for certain federal programs. 2018. https://aspe.hhs.gov/poverty-guidelines.
5. Baik CS, et al. Immuno-oncology clinical trial design: limitations, challenges, and opportunities. Clin Cancer Res. 2017;23:4992–5002. https://doi.org/10.1158/1078-0432.ccr-16-3066.
6. Bennette CS, Ramsey SD, McDermott CL, Carlson JJ, Basu A, Veenstra DL. Predicting low accrual in the National Cancer Institute's Cooperative Group Clinical Trials JNCI. J Natl Cancer Inst. 2016;108:djv324. https://doi.org/10.1093/jnci/djv324.
7. Bui Q, Sanger-Katz M. We mapped the uninsured. You'll notice a pattern. 2015. https://www.nytimes.com/interactive/2015/10/31/upshot/who-still-doesnt-have-health-insurance-obamacare.html.
8. Carrieri D, Peccatori FA, Boniolo G. The ethical plausibility of the 'Right To Try' laws. Crit Rev Oncol Hematol. 2018;122:64–71.
9. Center for Disease Control. National Center for Health Statistics FastStats: Centers for Disease Control and Prevention; 2017. https://www.cdc.gov/nchs/fastats/cancer.htm.
10. Census.gov. FFF: Older Americans month: May 2017 – Census.gov. 2017. https://www.census.gov/content/dam/Census/newsroom/facts-for-features/2017/cb17-ff08.pdf.
11. Cherubini A, Signore SD, Ouslander J, Semla T, Michel JP. Fighting against age discrimination in clinical trials. J Am Geriatr Soc. 2010;58:1791–6. https://doi.org/10.1111/j.1532-5415.2010.03032.x.
12. Clinicaltrials.gov. https://clinicaltrials.gov/ct2/results/map/click?recrs=a&type=Intr&cond=Breast+Cancer&cntry=US&age=12&phase=01234&mapw=1726&map.x=352&map.y=359. Accessed 4 June 2018.
13. Comarow A. FAQ: how and why we rank and rate hospitals. U.S. News & World Report. 2017. https://health.usnews.com/health-care/best-hospitals/articles/faq-how-and-why-we-rank-and-rate-hospitals. Accessed 14 June 2018.
14. DHEW. The Belmont report: ethical principles and guidelines for the protection of human subjects of research. 1979. https://www.hhs.gov/ohrp/sites/default/files/the-belmont-report-508c_FINAL.pdf.
15. Duma N, et al. Representation of minorities and women in oncology clinical trials: review of the past 14 years. J Oncol Pract. 2018;14:e1–e10. https://doi.org/10.1200/jop.2017.025288.
16. Elliott C. The anatomy of research scandals the Hastings Center Report 47:inside. 2017. https://doi.org/10.1002/hast.704.
17. Faden R, Kass N, Goodman S, Pronovost P, Tunis S, Beauchamp T. An ethics framework for a learning health care system: a departure from traditional research ethics and clinical ethics. Hastings Cent Rep. 2013;43:S16–27. https://doi.org/10.1002/hast.134.
18. Fayed L. Review of cost coverage for participating in a clinical trial. https://www.verywellhealth.com/are-clinical-trials-free-513637. Accessed 14 June 2018.
19. FDA 21 CFR 21 Part 56 Institutional Review Boards.
20. FDA 21 CFR 56.111 Criteria for IRB approval of research.
21. FDA. Guidance for industry: E9 statistical principles for clinical trials. 1998. https://www.fda.gov/downloads/drugs/guidancecomplianceregulatoryinformation/guidances/ucm073137.pdf.
22. FDA. 2004. IND exemptions for studies of lawfully marketed drug or biological products for the treatment of cancer. https://www.fda.gov/downloads/Drugs/GuidanceComplianceRegulatoryInformation/Guidances/UCM071717.pdf.

23. FDA. 2014. FDA action plan to enhance the collection and availability of demographic subgroup data. https://www.fda.gov/downloads/RegulatoryInformation/Legislation/FederalFood DrugandCosmeticActFDCAct/SignificantAmendmentstotheFDCAct/FDASIA/ UCM410474.pdf.

24. Ford I, Norrie J. Pragmatic trials. N Engl J Med. 2016;375:454–63. https://doi.org/10.1056/ NEJMra1510059.

25. Freedman RA, et al. Promoting accrual of older patients with cancer to clinical trials: an alliance for clinical trials in oncology member survey (A171602). Oncologist. 2018;23:1016. https://doi.org/10.1634/theoncologist.2018-0033.

26. Garcia S, et al. Thoracic oncology clinical trial eligibility criteria and requirements continue to increase in number and complexity. J Thorac Oncol. 2017;12:1489–95. https://doi. org/10.1016/j.jtho.2017.07.020.

27. Gerber DE, Lakoduk AM, Priddy LL, Yan J, Xie X-J. Temporal trends and predictors for cancer clinical trial availability for medically underserved populations. Oncologist. 2015;20:674–82. https://doi.org/10.1634/theoncologist.2015-0083.

28. Grady C. Payment of clinical research subjects. J Clin Invest. 2005;115:1681–7. https://doi. org/10.1172/JCI25694.

29. Gross CP, Krumholz HM, Van Wye G, Emanuel EJ, Wendler D. Does random treatment assignment cause harm to research participants? PLoS Med. 2006;3:e188.

30. Height DI. The need for justice in human participants research: life after the Belmont Commission. J Cancer Educ. 2009;24:S19. https://doi.org/10.1080/08858190903400401.

31. J. L. Semega, KR Fontenot, M.A. Kollar. Income and poverty in the United States: 2016 current population reports. 2017.

32. Jadhav S. Are clinical trial matching services truly patient-centric?. 2017. http://www.applied-clinicaltrialsonline.com/print/327315?page=full. Accessed 18 June 2018.

33. Jin S, Pazdur R, Sridhara R. Re-evaluating eligibility criteria for oncology clinical trials: analysis of investigational new drug applications in 2015. J Clin Oncol. 2017;35:3745–52. https://doi.org/10.1200/jco.2017.73.4186.

34. Joffe S, Weeks JC. Views of American oncologists about the purposes of clinical trials. J Natl Cancer Inst. 2002;94:1847–53. https://doi.org/10.1093/jnci/94.24.1847.

35. Johnson RG, Dornsife DL. Equitable access to cancer clinical trials: erasing the stigma of undue inducement. Oct 23, 2017. ASCO Connection. https://connection.asco.org/magazine/features/equitable-accesscancer-clinical-trials-erasing-stigma-undue-inducement.

36. Krohn T. Patient centricity in clinical trials: when searching is a struggle antidote. 2018. https://www.acrpnet.org/2018/01/17/patient-centricity-clinical-trials-searching-struggle/. Accessed 18 June 2018.

37. Lichtman SM, Hurria A, Jacobsen PB. Geriatric oncology: an overview. J Clin Oncol. 2014;32:2521–2. https://doi.org/10.1200/jco.2014.57.4822.

38. London A, Kimmelman J. Clinical trials in medical center advertising. JAMA Oncol. 2018;4:769. https://doi.org/10.1001/jamaoncol.2018.0181.

39. Manne S, et al. Attitudinal barriers to participation in oncology clinical trials: factor analysis and correlates of barriers. Eur J Cancer Care. 2015;24:28–38. https://doi.org/10.1111/ecc.12180.

40. Menikoff J, Kaneshiro J, Pritchard I. The common rule, updated. N Engl J Med. 2017;376:613–5. https://doi.org/10.1056/NEJMp1700736.

41. Murthy VH, Krumholz HM, Gross CP. Participation in cancer clinical trials: race-, sex-, and age-based disparities. JAMA. 2004;291:2720–6. https://doi.org/10.1001/jama.291.22.2720.

42. Narang AK, Nicholas L. Out-of-pocket spending and financial burden among medicare beneficiaries with cancer. JAMA Oncol. 2017;3:757–65. https://doi.org/10.1001/jamaoncol.2016.4865.

43. Nijjar S, D'Amico M, Wimalaweera N, Cooper N, Zamora J, Khan K. Participation in clinical trials improves outcomes in women's health: a systematic review and meta-analysis. BJOG. 2018;124:863–71. https://doi.org/10.1111/1471-0528.14528.. @10.1002/(ISSN)1471-0528(CAT)EditorsPick(VI)EditorsPick.

44. Nipp RD, et al. Financial burden of cancer clinical trial participation and the impact of a cancer care equity program. Oncologist. 2016;21:467–74. https://doi.org/10.1634/theoncologist.2015-0481.
45. Right to Try Movement. 2018. http://righttotry.org/. Accessed 13 June 2018.
46. Siegel RL, Miller KD, Jemal A. Cancer statistics, 2017. CA Cancer J Clin. 2017;67:7–30. https://doi.org/10.3322/caac.21387.
47. Singh GK, Jemal A. Socioeconomic and racial/ethnic disparities in cancer mortality, incidence, and survival in the United States, 1950-2014: over six decades of changing patterns and widening inequalities. J Environ Public Health. 2017;2017:2819372. https://doi.org/10.1155/2017/2819372.
48. Strauss DC, Thomas JM. What does the medical profession mean by "Standard of Care?". J Clin Oncol. 2009;27:e192–3. https://doi.org/10.1200/jco.2009.24.6678.
49. Townsley CA, Selby R, Siu LL. Systematic review of barriers to the recruitment of older patients with cancer onto clinical trials. J Clin Oncol. 2005;23:3112–24. https://doi.org/10.1200/jco.2005.00.141.
50. Unger JM, Gralow JR, Albain KS, Ramsey SD, Hershman DL. Patient income level and cancer clinical trial participation: a prospective survey study. JAMA Oncol. 2016;2:137–9. https://doi.org/10.1001/jamaoncol.2015.3924.
51. Wallach JD, Ross JS, Naci H. The US Food and Drug Administration's expedited approval programs: evidentiary standards, regulatory trade-offs, and potential improvements. Clin Trials. 2018;15:219–29. https://doi.org/10.1177/1740774518770648.
52. Weber JS, et al. American Society of Clinical Oncology policy statement update: the critical role of phase I trials in cancer research and treatment. J Clin Oncol. 2015;33:278–84. https://doi.org/10.1200/jco.2014.58.2635.
53. Wong Y-N, et al. Financial concerns about participation in clinical trials among patients with cancer. J Clin Oncol. 2016;34:479–87. https://doi.org/10.1200/jco.2015.63.2463.

Chapter 6
Global Disparities: Can the World Afford Cancer?

Haydee Cristina Verduzco-Aguirre, Enrique Soto-Perez-de-Celis, Yanin Chavarri-Guerra, and Gilberto Lopes

Introduction

The last few decades have brought significant breakthroughs in the treatment of cancer, which have led to an improvement in the outcomes of patients worldwide. However, access to these treatments is limited for patients living in low-and-middle-income countries (LMICs) or in resource-limited settings in high-income countries (HICs). According to data from GLOBOCAN, in 2012 there were 14.1 million new cases of cancer and 8.2 million cancer deaths across the world. Strikingly, 57% of those new cancer cases and 65% of cancer-related deaths occurred in LMICs, where healthcare systems are less prepared to treat noncommunicable diseases such as cancer. This is easily demonstrable by analyzing the mortality-to-incidence ratio (MIR) across different regions of the world. The aggregate MIR for all types of cancer in more developed regions of the world, for example, is 0.475 (which means that 47.5% of patients diagnosed with cancer will eventually die from the disease), whereas in less developed regions, the MIR is of 0.664, representing an almost 20% higher chance of dying after a diagnosis of cancer [21]. Wide differences in cancer-specific outcomes, such as 5-year overall survival (OS), are also found between

H. C. Verduzco-Aguirre · Y. Chavarri-Guerra
Department of Hemato-Oncology, Instituto Nacional de Ciencias Médicas y Nutrición
Salvador Zubirán, Tlalpan, Mexico City, Mexico

E. Soto-Perez-de-Celis
Department of Geriatrics, Instituto Nacional de Ciencias Médicas y Nutrición Salvador
Zubirán, Tlalpan, Mexico City, Mexico

G. Lopes (✉)
Sylvester Comprehensive Cancer Center, University of Miami and the Miller School
of Medicine, Miami, FL, USA
e-mail: glopes@med.miami.edu

© Springer Nature Switzerland AG 2019
E. H. Bernicker (ed.), *Cancer and Society*,
https://doi.org/10.1007/978-3-030-05855-5_6

LMICs and HICs. Five-year age-standardized net survival rates for breast cancer (all stages) in the period comprised between 2010 and 2014, for example, were of 90.2% in the United States and 86.7% in France, compared with 75.2% in Brazil, 68.7% in Thailand, and only 40.1% in South Africa [2].

The incidence of cancer is estimated to continue rising during the following decades, with a global increase of around 70% by the year 2035, and this rise is expected to be higher in LMICs [21]). There are many reasons for this increase in cancer incidence in LMIC, but one of its main drivers is that these countries are still completing their demographic transition, which will lead to an increase in the number of older adults, which are at higher risk of developing cancer – in fact, the largest increase in incidence is predicted in people older than 65 years of age, with an increase of over 100% in new cancer cases. Another potential reason for the increased cancer incidence in LMICs is an increasing exposure to risk factors, such as tobacco use and obesity, which are greatly prevalent in many LMICs [37].

Healthcare Expenditure and Cancer Care

Despite this growing global burden of cancer, many healthcare systems are not well prepared to manage this epidemiological transition. This is an even greater issue in LMICs, since it has been estimated that only 5% of the global resources for cancer control are spent in these countries [20].

Government Investment in Healthcare

While all regions of the world will see an increase in cancer, there are large differences among countries regarding expenditure on health, which depends both on gross domestic product per capita (GDP) and on the percentage of GDP allocated to healthcare. These differences can be seen between HICs and LMICs but also within different LMICs. In 2014, for example, Kenya (a lower-middle-income country according to the World Bank) spent 169 USD per capita on healthcare, corresponding to 5.7% of the country's GDP. In that same year, Mexico, an upper-middle-income country, spent 1122–1318 USD (6.3–8.3% of GDP), while a HIC like Canada spent $4641 per capita (10.4% of GDP) [55]. The annual economic burden of cancer per patient, including direct medical expenses (procedures, hospitalizations, outpatient visits, and prescription drugs), nonmedical expenses (transportation and caregiving), and productivity losses, has been calculated in a range from 0.54 to 7.92 USD in developing regions such as South America, China, and India. In comparison, HICs such as the United Kingdom (UK), Japan, and the United States (US) spend 183–460 USD per patient. Translating this to per capita gross national income (GNI), expenditure on cancer care is equivalent to 0.05–0.12% of GNI in developing regions such as South America, China, and India. In contrast, these expenses correspond to 0.51–1.02% of GNI in HIC [30].

There are also great variations in financing of cancer care across countries, with different proportions of government contributions and household out-of-pocket expenses. Although this happens in every region, a larger proportion of the population of LMICs is exposed to potentially catastrophic out-of-pocket expenditure. This is partially due to the existence of fragmented healthcare systems with limited coverage for expensive conditions such as cancer. In Mexico, for example, there are at least six different public healthcare systems, with each having different availability of treatments and procedures [44].

Access to Cancer Medications, and Affordability of Cancer Care

A fundamental issue that must be taken into account when analyzing the global affordability of cancer care is the cost of medications. Global spending on cancer therapies and supportive care drugs now exceeds 133 billion USD, and this expenditure will continue increasing, with a projected 180–200 billion USD spent in cancer drugs globally during the next 5 years [27]. Spending on cancer medications has increased steadily for the last 10 years, in parallel with a rise in list prices of newer drugs. These increases have been particularly steep since the introduction of newer classes of drugs, such as checkpoint inhibitors and targeted agents. The median annual cost of a new cancer drug launched in 2014 exceeded 135,000 USD, representing approximately 6 times the cost of cancer drugs approved in the early 2000s, after adjusting for inflation [16]. More recently, personalized cell-based therapies, such as chimeric antigen receptor (CAR) T-cell immunotherapy, are listed at an even higher price of around 375–475,000 USD per patient [15].

These high costs represent a major barrier to access for patients in LMICs. The very definition of LMIC implies a GNI per capita of $12,235, many times less than the cost of some of the newer medications as single agents [54]. For many patients, this can mean incurring in catastrophic out-of-pocket expenses and, for many others, simply not having access to medications. Moreover, when LMIC try to provide newer therapies as part of public healthcare coverage, their cost can take over a large proportion of the total cancer-related expenditure. A good example of this is Lebanon, where in 2016 pembrolizumab and nivolumab represented 19% of the total yearly budget for cancer medications, despite only being used for 3% of all patients with cancer in the country [18]. Therefore, national healthcare policy makers need to prioritize which interventions and medications have the largest potential benefit at the lowest possible cost. However, with the large number of cancer drugs launched every year, and national differences in availability and access, this can be very difficult to outline.

The World Health Organization (WHO) has previously published the Model List of Essential Medicines, which includes a section on essential cancer medications.

This list was recently updated in 2015 in conjunction with the Union for International Cancer Control (UICC). Cancer care specialists from all continents participated in this value-oriented review, identifying cancer types with potential for maximal treatment impact. The value of individual systemic agents was assessed based on incidence, treatment outcomes (including all therapeutic options such as surgery, radiotherapy, and systemic agents), and absolute and relative benefit of available systemic therapies. This update resulted in 16 medications added to the list, compared to the last update in 1999. It is important to highlight that only three of the drugs in the current list can be considered as high-cost medications: imatinib, trastuzumab, and rituximab. Also, none of the drugs included in the list were launched or approved after 2010 [43] (Table 6.1).

It must be noted as well that this list remains only a guide and does not compel individual countries to provide any of the included medications. In fact, an analysis of 135 national essential or reimbursable medicine lists performed in 2015 showed that only 48% of WHO recommended medications were included on average [40]. This varied among income groups, with lists from low-income countries including an average of only 10 of the essential cancer medications, compared to an average of 30 for HICs [46].

One of the newly added drugs, trastuzumab, is included in the list only in the context of early-stage breast cancer. This is justified by breast cancer being highly prevalent and potentially curable at these stages and by the fact that trastuzumab administered for 1 year increases survival from 75.2% to 84.0% when added to standard chemotherapy [36]. Importantly, trastuzumab's entry in the WHO list also includes as a requirement the performance of hormone receptor analysis by immunohistochemistry (IHC) and HER2 evaluation by IHC or fluorescence in situ hybridization, in order to clearly identify candidates for HER2-targeted therapy. Trastuzumab has been shown to be cost-effective in HICs such as Europe and Singapore [11, 50], although there is a lack of information regarding its cost-effectiveness in LMICs.

Adding more systemic agents can lead to increasing cure rates but, as expected, it may also result in higher treatment costs. As an example, while addition of rituximab to standard CHOP chemotherapy (cyclophosphamide, doxorubicin, vincristine, and prednisone) for diffuse large B-cell lymphoma increases the cure rate from 55% to more than 70%, this also increases the cost of treatment from approximately 200 to 6000 USD for 6 cycles of therapy (without including additional costs from administration of therapy). However, a large magnitude of benefit is obtained by the addition of rituximab alone, and this was the basis for its inclusion in the updated WHO Essential Medicines List [43].

It is also worth noting that the high cost of newer drugs does not always translate into clinically meaningful and/or cost-effective improvements in outcomes. As a matter of fact, between 2008 and 2012 the US Food and Drugs Administration (FDA) approved 36 uses for cancer drugs without evidence of benefit in OS or quality of life (QoL), representing 67% of the approvals during that time period [38]. In

Table 6.1 World Health Organization Essential Medicines List for cancer medications

Essential drugs	
Antineoplastic and adjuvant	Hormones and antihormones
All-trans-retinoic acid[b]	Anastrozole[b]
Allopurinol	Bicalutamide[b]
Asparaginase	Dexamethasone
Bendamustine[a,b]	Leuprorelin[a,b]
Bleomycin	Hydrocortisone
Calcium folinate	Methylprednisolone
Capecitabine[b]	Prednisolone
Carboplatin	Tamoxifen
Chlorambucil	
Cisplatin[b]	
Cyclophosphamide	
Cytarabine	
Dacarbazine	
Dactinomycin	
Daunorubicin	
Docetaxel	
Doxorubicin	
Etoposide	
Fludarabine[b]	
Fluorouracil	
Filgrastim[b]	
Gemcitabine[b]	
Hydroxycarbamide	
Ifosfamide	
Imatinib[a,b]	
Irinotecan[b]	
Mercaptopurine	
Mesna	
Methotrexate	
Oxaliplatin[b]	
Procarbazine	
Rituximab[a,b]	
Tioguanine	
Trastuzumab[a,b]	
Vinblastine	
Vincristine	
Vinorelbine	

[a]On patent in the United States and/or the European Union
[b]Added in 2015

non-small cell lung cancer (NSCLC), for example, the use of newer drugs has made the average cost per patient rise about fourfold since 2000, but five-year OS is still less than 10% [52]. In fact, two drugs used to treat NSCLC harboring epidermal growth factor receptor (EGFR) mutations, erlotinib and gefitinib, were not accepted for the update of 2015 WHO Essential Medicines List. The main justification for their exclusion was that the impact of therapy was relatively modest (prolongation of progression-free survival [PFS] by 3–4 months). However, there were also infrastructural and financial concerns surrounding the availability of reliable molecular testing for EGFR mutations, which could have hampered their correct use in limited-resource settings [46]. Regardless of their exclusion from the list, analyses performed in Spain, France, and Italy have shown that erlotinib may be cost-effective when compared to chemotherapy for first-line treatment of EGFR-mutated NSCLC [51]. These results have also been reproduced in Asian patients in China, and it is likely that future editions of the list may include EGFR-targeting agents once the tools to perform mutation testing are more widely available [53].

So, what makes newer drugs considerably more expensive? One of the most prevalent arguments to justify this is the great investment made in the phases of drug development. An analysis from the Tufts Center for the Study of Drug Development estimated that it costs 2.7 billion USD (adjusted for inflation in 2017) to bring a single drug into the US market [14]. These figures, however, have been contested by other analyses. Public Citizen, a nonprofit advocacy group, estimated that $320 million were needed to develop a new cancer drug [57]. Another analysis, using the US Securities and Exchange Commission filings for 10 cancer drugs approved between 2006 and 2015, reported that the median cost of developing a single cancer drug was $648.0 million, with a range from $157.3 million to $1950.8 million. This analysis took into account expenses for research and development of other failed drugs by the same pharmaceutical companies. At a median time since approval of 4 years, the median revenue for each of these 10 drugs was $1658.4 million, ranging between $204.1 million and $22275.0 million. Mean length of market exclusivity for cancer drugs is 14.3 years, so it is expected that the reported revenues will continue to increase over time [39].

Access to Radiation Therapy

Between 50% and 60% of patients with cancer will require radiation therapy at some point of their disease trajectory [13]. Ensuring access to radiation therapy can lead to improvements in treatment outcomes and QoL, since this treatment modality is used throughout all stages of the natural history of cancer. Unfortunately, there are wide disparities in access and affordability of radiotherapy around the world, and only about half of patients are estimated to have access to radiation therapy globally. The current cost of a radiation therapy course is around 1226–6581 USD, which translates to a cost per treatment fraction ranging from 60 to 363 USD, with the lowest costs in Africa and the highest in Europe and North America. These costs depend mostly on equipment utilization rate and maintenance costs [59].

There is an enormous need to improve global access to radiotherapy, both for curative-intent treatments and for palliation of symptoms such as pain or bleeding. In Africa, for example, equipment is unevenly distributed: data from 2013 reported that over 60% of radiotherapy machines were located in Egypt and South Africa, whereas 29 of 54 African countries lacked any radiotherapy machine [25]. In order to provide adequate coverage to African patients, there is a need to approximately double the current number of cancer centers, radiotherapy units, and trained staff [59]. However, an increase in the number of radiotherapy units needs to be coupled with an appropriate distribution of treatment centers across national territories. Currently, even in countries with adequate or almost-adequate resources, most radiotherapy-capable hospitals are located in large cities, and patients living in rural regions have to travel long distances to receive treatment [4]. Additionally, the quality of available radiotherapy services is questionable, and many centers in developing countries utilize outdated machines, placing patients at risk of worse toxicities and poor outcomes. In Latin America, for example, a considerable proportion of radiotherapy centers lack simulation or treatment-planning systems [58].

Availability of Preventive Strategies

A significant proportion of cancer in LMICs is infection-related and thus potentially preventable through immunization or eradication of microorganisms. Both cervical cancer and hepatocellular carcinoma are mostly caused by viruses, which are potentially preventable through vaccination. Currently, WHO guidelines recommend vaccination against hepatitis B virus (HBV) at birth and against human papillomavirus (HPV) for girls aged 9–14 [56].

Unfortunately, coverage of vaccination for these potentially preventable diseases is limited. The worldwide coverage of HPV vaccination among 10–20-year-old women, for example, is of only about 6%. Coverage is lower among women living in LMIC in Africa and Asia, with only 1% of eligible women vaccinated as of 2014 [7]. Barriers to the uptake of HPV vaccination include inadequate financing and health infrastructure, provider reluctance to recommend the vaccine, and rumors about vaccination-related adverse events [22].

Increasing the coverage of HPV vaccination could have profound effects on cancer control. With a global coverage of 90%, for instance, between 443,000 to 690,000 cervical cancer cases and 229,000 to 420,000 cervical cancer-related deaths could be averted [49]. Importantly, this benefit would be larger in LMICs, where most of the cases are concentrated. Additionally, bivalent HPV vaccination has been shown to be cost-effective in most countries [28].

Improving Global Access to Cancer Care

International organizations, such as the United Nations (UN), have highlighted global cancer control as one of their highest priorities. The UN 2030 Agenda for Sustainable Development includes two cancer-related targets: first, the reduction in premature mortality from NCDs, including cancer, by one-third by 2030, and, second, the achievement of universal health coverage, including financial risk protection, access to quality essential healthcare service, and access to effective, quality, and affordable essential medicines and vaccines for all [47].

Role of National Governments

People living in LMICs face substantial financial vulnerabilities when diagnosed with cancer. In India, for example, the cost of a single hospital admission due to cancer-related morbidity at a public hospital is the equivalent of 40–50% of the per capita GDP [32]. These catastrophic expenses often force patients and their families to incur in borrowing or selling their assets to finance treatments. Out-of-pocket spending is one of the two primary sources of financing of cancer care in LMICs (mostly at point of care, rarely via private insurance), the other being public spending for health or social protection in the fashion of public insurance. According to data from the World Bank, out-of-pocket expenditure constituted 36.6% of all healthcare costs in LMICs in 2015, compared to 13.5% in HICs [54].

In order to protect people from financial hardship and out-of-pocket catastrophic expenses that would preclude them from obtaining needed healthcare services, some LMICs are slowly transitioning to providing universal health coverage. However, in some cases universal health coverage may not be of optimal quality. In Mexico, for example, the *Seguro Popular* public insurance system was created in 2003 to provide healthcare coverage to a sector of the population who was previously uninsured, mostly due to a lack of formal employment. While *Seguro Popular* has progressively expanded its portfolio of covered drugs and interventions, only eight types of cancer are currently covered for adults and, even for those tumor types, not all available interventions and treatments are covered (including newer drugs, treatment of adverse events leading to hospitalization, and palliative care) [44, 10].

A fundamental step for selecting the most appropriate and cost-effective treatments and interventions to cover is to understand local epidemiology. In order to achieve this very important goal, all countries should have a cancer registry to serve as guidance for healthcare planning. Despite progress in recent years, most LMICs still do not have proper population-based cancer registries. Only nine low-to-medium Human Development Index countries (China, Egypt, India, Malawi, Philippines, South Africa, Thailand, Uganda, and Zimbabwe) have high-quality population-based cancer registries, all of which have only regional coverage. Without proper information about the national cancer burden, countries are unable to allocate scarce resources adequately and efficiently [3]. Additionally, the development of cancer registries goes hand in hand with the establishment of national cancer control plans (NCCP) including interventions throughout all the stages of cancer care (research and development, primary prevention, diagnosis, treatment, and palliative care). Some regions of the world have made progress toward establishing NCCP, even in the absence of cancer registries. In Latin America, for example, there was an 8% increase in the number of countries with a NCCP between 2011 and 2014 and, as of 2014, 60% of the countries in the region possessed a NCCP [12, 44].

Role of International Organizations and Trade Regulations

International organizations and governing bodies have an essential role in the achievement of affordable and universal cancer care. At the same time, some international regulations also represent barriers in access to therapies in developing countries. World Trade Organization (WTO)-affiliated countries, for example, are required by the Trade-Related Aspects of Intellectual Property Rights (TRIPS) agreement to provide patent protection for medications for at least 20 years, in order to protect intellectual property of pharmaceutical and other products. In order to make it possible for developing countries to gain access to novel, potentially lifesaving therapies, WTO issued the 2001 Doha Declaration, which provided countries the capacity to issue compulsory licenses for drugs considered essential for public health. Compulsory licensing allows healthcare systems in resource-limited countries to circumvent patent laws and to allow production of generic versions of patent-protected drugs. The Doha Declaration also allows LMICs to import medications produced in countries under compulsory licensing. This mechanism has been widely used to gain access to medications targeting infectious diseases, such as HIV, hepatitis C, tuberculosis, and malaria. Compulsory licenses for cancer medications, however, have not been as widely used in LMICs. Only India (sorafenib), Thailand (docetaxel, letrozole, and erlotinib), and Ecuador (sorafenib) have used compulsory licensing in order to ensure access to cancer drugs. Even when compulsory licenses are denied, the sole pursuing of this legal resource has pressured some companies such as Roche, who abandoned its patent claims for trastuzumab after India pursued a compulsory license for this drug [31]. In some other cases, the threat of compulsory licensing may make pharmaceutical companies offer more affordable prices when acquiring medications in bulk [5]. Critics of compulsory licensing argue that it decreases incentives for innovation, although evidence for this is scarce, since the largest portion of revenue for cancer drugs comes from HICs. In some cases, the pharmaceutical industry has pressured countries to discourage them from compulsory licensing, for example, by threatening to retire local investments [1]. However, even in the absence of international pressure, many countries are unable to issue compulsory licenses due to a lack of adequate legislation to pursue it.

International organizations can also improve access to cancer care through the development of partnerships with local governments and stakeholders, leading to capacity building and provision of equipment. An example of this is the Program of Action for Cancer Therapy (PACT) developed by the International Atomic Energy Agency (IAEA). Through PACT, a comprehensive assessment of local needs is undertaken, a full team of local healthcare providers receives training, and equipment is procured via cost-sharing agreements between IAEA and local governments [41].

Generic and Biosimilar Medications

When patents expire, companies can start developing generic versions of medications, which may lead to price drops of around 80% or more [9]. However, there is a lack of information regarding the economic impact of generic drugs in oncology, be it in high- or low-resource settings. In India, for example, generic paclitaxel, docetaxel, gemcitabine, oxaliplatin, and irinotecan have been estimated to provide potential cost savings of almost 843 million USD [29]. However, there are still some concerns regarding the efficacy and safety of many generic drugs, which may hamper their utilization by oncologists. Quality manufacturing and supervision by regulatory agencies is therefore an essential part of the development of generic drugs in order to confirm their bioequivalence to their branded versions [29].

As previously stated, biologics are among the most expensive cancer drugs, in part due to complex manufacturing processes. In the last few years, biosimilars, which are almost identical products to the originator biologic drug, have emerged as an option to biologics. Several antineoplastic biosimilars have started or completed their development, as several biologics will lose their patents in the coming years. The largest manufacturers of biosimilars reside in the United States, Europe, and Israel but also in LMICs such as India, China, and Brazil [9]. The approval of biosimilars requires demonstration of similarity in pharmacokinetics, efficacy, safety, and immunogenicity. The first biosimilar approved by the EMA was somatropin in 2006, while the FDA approved biosimilar filgrastim-sndz in 2015. Other FDA-approved biosimilars include bevacizumab-awwb, trastuzumab-dkst, and pegfilgrastim-jmdb. Additionally, India has approved biosimilar rituximab [48, 19].

Biosimilars are currently sold at about 30–70% less than the cost of the originator drug, which could bring important cost savings in biologic-related expenses. Still, some challenges remain for the widespread adoption of biosimilars. Selecting adequate endpoints for similarity studies is still a point of debate, although surrogate endpoints such as objective response rate are acceptable according to EMA guidelines. Another subject of discussion is if extrapolation to all approved indications of a biologic drug is possible with a biosimilar study conducted only on one indication. Safety concerns related to immunogenicity or difference in adverse events due to minor changes are also a concern, which would require strict quality control during the manufacturing process. Lastly, but equally important, knowledge regarding biosimilars remains relatively low among both healthcare providers and patients [9].

Alternative Strategies to Improve Access to Novel Therapies

An alternative to compulsory licensing is price discrimination, also called tiered pricing. Price discrimination means selling identical goods or services at different prices in different markets, depending on the ability and willingness to pay of the customer. Some pharmaceutical companies have recently introduced price discrimination for cancer drugs in different global markets [5]. However, price discrimination could potentially lead to parallel imports to HIC from LMICs with lower drug prices and create a political backlash [29].

In some cases, pharmaceutical companies have established expanded access programs. An example of this is Novartis' Glivec International Patient Assistance Program (GIPAP), which has provided around 2.3 million monthly doses of imatinib to more than 49,000 patients with Philadelphia-chromosome positive chronic myeloid leukemia or with c-Kit positive unresectable and/or metastatic gastrointestinal stromal tumors (GIST) in 81 developing countries [23]. A similar program has been developed by Gavi, the Vaccine Alliance, a public-private partnership aimed at increasing access to new and underused vaccines for children living in developing countries. Gavi's actions have led to an increased uptake of HPV vaccination in various LMICs through temporary demonstration projects or deep discounts. However, not all pilot programs have led to the development of national vaccination strategies [6].

Creating the Evidence Base for Reducing Drug Pricing

The oncologic scientific community, in conjunction with pharmaceutical companies, has an essential role in lowering the cost of cancer care. One way in which basic and clinical investigators can harness research to reduce the cost of cancer care is by developing more effective biomarkers. Biomarkers can improve patient selection for both clinical trials and real-world clinical practice and lead to a better characterization of subgroups which might benefit the most from newer therapies. A good example of the appropriate use of biomarkers for drug development is NSCLC, where the use of biomarkers such as EGFR or programmed death ligand 1 (PD-L1) has improved the selection of patients who might benefit from costly treatments such as immunotherapy. For example, in patients with metastatic NSCLC and a tumor proportion score for PD-L1 of $\geq 1\%$, the cost/life-year gain of pembrolizumab is 659,059 USD, while in those with a PD-L1 score of $\geq 50\%$, it is only 186,897 USD. In this case, the use of a biomarker may lead to an improved and more cost-effective selection of patients who might benefit the most from a costly therapy [26].

Cancer care providers, such as physicians and non-physician clinical staff, have a central role in promoting access to medications. Physicians must be able to analyze current evidence, present it to the patient, and select the best treatment options in the context of shared decision-making. In order to help clinicians choose wisely among the myriad of new cancer therapies, several international organizations have developed frameworks to assess the value of treatments. The European Society of Medical Oncology's (ESMO) Magnitude of Clinical Benefit Scale is a validated tool that can be applied to stratify the benefits of solid cancer treatments, both in curative and palliative settings [8]. The American Society of Clinical Oncology's (ASCO) Value Framework also focuses on clinical benefit, toxicity, and symptom palliation, combining them to obtain a score termed "net health benefit" [42]. Additionally, the Drug Pricing Lab at Memorial Sloan Kettering Cancer Center has created DrugAbacus, a tool that provides estimates of value-based prices. By its calculations, almost 80% of cancer drugs in the United States cost more than their value-based price [33]. These tools provide a more objective way to compare the benefits and cost-effectiveness of currently available therapies.

A valuable tool for clinicians practicing in resource-limited setting is the use of resource-stratified guidelines. Resource-stratified guidelines were first proposed by the Breast Health Global Initiative, and both ASCO and the National Comprehensive Cancer Network (NCCN) followed their lead in order to provide frameworks for identifying essential therapies and procedures for each level of available resources (basic, limited, enhanced, and maximal). These frameworks have been created in conjunction with clinicians who regularly practice in resource-limited settings, as well as policy makers [35]. Using this information, oncologists can adapt their practice according to the local resource environment, whether they have basic, limited, or enhanced tools at their disposal, and offer treatments with the greatest value to their patients.

Clinical researchers can also improve access to expensive therapies by designing innovative clinical trials aimed at increasing the value of treatments. One potential strategy to achieve this is the use of shorter treatment durations of expensive medications. An example of this strategy is the recently presented PERSEPHONE randomized controlled trial (RCT), which demonstrated that 6 months of adjuvant trastuzumab was noninferior to the standard 12 months of therapy in terms of disease-free survival, albeit at a lesser cost and with less cardiotoxicity [17]. Modifications in dosing could potentially also lead to cost savings, particularly for high-priced drugs like immunotherapy. A recently published pharmacoeconomic analysis showed that using a personalized (2 mg/kg) dosing of pembrolizumab instead of the currently approved fixed dose (200 mg) for patients with NSCLC could potentially save 0.825 billion USD in the United States alone [24]. A third potential strategy is modifying drug pharmacokinetics using simple interventions, such as administering drugs with food rather than on an empty stomach. This premise was tested in a small phase II study in patients with prostate cancer receiving abiraterone. In that study, a 250 mg dose of abiraterone taken with a low-fat meal was shown to be noninferior to the standard 1000 mg dose, with the primary outcome being a logarithmic change in prostate-specific antigen (PSA). At a cost of approximately $10,000 per month, per-patient cost savings would range from $100,000 for metastatic castration-resistant prostate cancer to more than $300,000 for metastatic castration-sensitive prostate cancer [45]. Unfortunately, a barrier to this type of studies is the lack of funding, since pharmaceutical companies may not be interested in financing them. Therefore, governmental organizations should make it a priority to provide funding to studies aiming at increasing the value of drugs. An encouraging example of this is the fact that the aforementioned PERSEPHONE RCT study was funded by the Health Technology Assessment arm of the National Institute for Health Research in the UK.

Lastly, cooperation between public and private organizations is essential. Patient advocacy groups historically have been able to influence policy makers, such as in the case of AIDS activism. In Brazil, for example, *Instituto Oncoguia* (a nonprofit organization representing people living with cancer) campaigned on mass media to pressure the government into including oral anticancer medicines in public health insurance coverage, ultimately succeeding [34].

Conclusion

Improving global access to cancer care requires a coordinated effort at all levels: regional and local institutions and governments, international organizations, pharmaceutical companies, healthcare providers, researchers, and patient organizations. In order for the world to afford cancer care, healthcare systems, policy makers, and physicians must be proficient in the assessment of the value and cost-effectiveness of current treatments, including chemotherapy, targeted therapies, radiation therapy, surgery, and preventive measures such as vaccination. Ultimately, our goal must be to ensure access to essential lifesaving, life-prolonging medications and to help patients make decisions that will provide the best possible outcomes, regardless of their setting.

References

1. Allam A. Seeking Investment, Egypt Tries Patent Laws, The New York Times. 2002. Available at: https://www.nytimes.com/2002/10/04/business/seeking-investment-egypt-tries-patent-laws.html.
2. Allemani C, Matsuda T, Di Carlo V, Harewood R, Matz M, Nikšić M, Bonaventure A, Valkov M, Johnson CJ, Estève J, Ogunbiyi OJ, Azevedo E, Silva G, Chen WQ, Eser S, Engholm G, Stiller CA, Monnereau A, Woods RR, Visser O, Lim GH, Aitken J, Weir HK, Coleman MP, CONCORD Working Group. Global surveillance of trends in cancer survival 2000-14 (CONCORD-3): analysis of individual records for 37 513 025 patients diagnosed with one of 18 cancers from 322 population-based registries in 71 countries. Lancet. 2018;391(10125):1023–75.
3. American Cancer Society. Cancer registries. The surveillance of cancer. Cancer Atlas. 2014. Available at: http://canceratlas.cancer.org/. Accessed 28 June 2018.
4. Atun R, Jaffray DA, Barton MB, Bray F, Baumann M, Vikram B, Hanna TP, Knaul FM, Lievens Y, Lui TY, Milosevic M, O'Sullivan B, Rodin DL, Rosenblatt E, Van Dyk J, Yap ML, Zubizarreta E, Gospodarowicz M. Expanding global access to radiotherapy. Lancet Oncol. 2015;16(10):1153–86.

5. Bognar CLFB, Bychkovsky BL, Lopes GL. Compulsory licenses for cancer drugs: does circumventing patent rights improve access to oncology medications? J Glob Oncol. 2016;2(5):292–301.
6. Botwright S, Holroyd T, Nanda S, Bloem P, Griffiths UK, Sidibe A, Hutubessy RCW. Experiences of operational costs of HPV vaccine delivery strategies in Gavi-supported demonstration projects. PLoS One. 2017;12(10):e0182663.
7. Bruni L, Diaz M, Barrionuevo-Rosas L, Herrero R, Bray F, Bosch FX, de Sanjosé S, Castellsagué X. Global estimates of human papillomavirus vaccination coverage by region and income level: a pooled analysis. Lancet Glob Health. 2016;4(7):e453–63.
8. Cherny NI, Dafni U, Bogaerts J, Latino NJ, Pentheroudakis G, Douillard JY, Tabernero J, Zielinski C, Piccart MJ, de Vries EGE. ESMO-magnitude of clinical benefit scale version 1.1. Ann Oncol. 2017;28(10):2340–66.
9. Chopra R, Lopes G. Improving access to cancer treatments: the role of biosimilars. J Glob Oncol. 2017;3(5):596–610.
10. Comision Nacional de Proteccion Social en Salud. Intervenciones del fondo de proteccion contra gastos catastroficos. 2018; http://www.seguropopularcolima.gob.mx/segpop/pdf/inter-vencionesGastosCatastroficos.pdf (Accessed 28 Dec 2018).
11. de Lima Lopes G. Societal costs and benefits of treatment with trastuzumab in patients with early HER2neu-overexpressing breast cancer in Singapore. BMC Cancer. 2011;11:178.
12. de Souza JA, Hunt B, Asirwa FC, Adebamowo C, Lopes G. Global health equity: cancer care outcome disparities in high-, middle-, and low-income countries. J Clin Oncol. 2016;34(1):6–13.
13. Delaney GP, Barton MB. Evidence-based estimates of the demand for radiotherapy. Clin Oncol (R Coll RAdiol). 2015;27(2):70–6.
14. DiMasi JA, Grabowski HG, Hansen RW. Innovation in the pharmaceutical industry: new esti-mates of R&D costs. J Health Econ. 2016;47:20–33.
15. Dolgin E. Bringing down the cost of cancer treatment. Nature. 2018;555(7695):S26–9.
16. Dusetzina SB. Drug pricing trends for orally administered anticancer medications reimbursed by commercial health plans, 2000–2014. JAMA Oncol. 2016;2(7):960–1.
17. Earl HM, Hiller L, Vaillier A-L, Dunn J, et al. PERSEPHONE: 6 versus 12 months (m) of adjuvant trastuzumab in patients (pts) with HER2 positive (+) early breast cancer (EBC): ran-domised phase 3 non-inferiority trial with definitive 4-year (yr) disease-free survival (DFS) results. J Clin Oncol. 2018;36(15_suppl):506.
18. Elias F, Bou-Orm IR, Adib SM, Gebran S, Gebran A, Ammar W. Cost of oncology drugs in the middleeastern country of Lebanon: an update (2014–2016). J Glob Oncol. 2018;(4):1–7.
19. European Medicines Agency. European public assessment reports – biosimilars. Available at: http://www.ema.europa.eu/ema/index.jsp?curl=pages/medicines/landing/epar_search.jsp&mid=WC0b01ac058001d124. Accessed 28 June 2018.
20. Farmer P, Frenk J, Knaul FM, Shulman LN, Alleyne G, Armstrong L, Atun R, Blayney D, Chen L, Feachem R, Gospodarowicz M, Gralow J, Gupta S, Langer A, Lob-Levyt J, Neal C, Mbewu A, Mired D, Piot P, Reddy KS, Sachs JD, Sarhan M, Seffrin JR. Expansion of cancer care and control in countries of low and middle income: a call to action. Lancet. 2010;376(9747):1186–93.
21. Ferlay J, Soerjomataram I, Dikshit R, Eser S, Mathers C, Rebelo M, Parkin DM, Forman D, Bray F. Cancer incidence and mortality worldwide: sources, methods and major patterns in GLOBOCAN 2012. Int J Cancer. 2015;136(5):E359–86.
22. Gallagher KE, LaMontagne DS, Watson-Jones D. Status of HPV vaccine introduction and barriers to country uptake. Vaccine. 2018;36(32 Pt A):4761–7.
23. Garcia-Gonzalez P, Boultbee P, Epstein D. Novel Humanitarian Aid Program: the Glivec International Patient Assistance Program-lessons learned from providing access to break-through targeted oncology treatment in low- and middle-income countries. J Glob Oncol. 2015;1(1):37–45.
24. Goldstein DA, Gordon N, Davidescu M, Leshno M, Steuer CE, Patel N, Stemmer SM, Zer A. A phamacoeconomic analysis of personalized dosing vs fixed dosing of pembrolizumab

in firstline PD-L1-positive non-small cell lung cancer. J Natl Cancer Inst. 2017;109(11) https://doi.org/10.1093/jnci/djx063.

25. Grover S, Xu MJ, Yeager A, Rosman L, Groen RS, Chackungal S, Rodin D, Mangaali M, Nurkic S, Fernandes A, Lin LL, Thomas G, Tergas AI. A systematic review of radiotherapy capacity in low- and middle-income countries. Front Oncol. 2014;4:380.

26. Guirgis HM. The impact of PD-L1 on survival and value of the immune check point inhibitors in non-small-cell lung cancer; proposal, policies and perspective. J Immunother Cancer. 2018;6(1):15.

27. IQVIA Institute for Human Data Science. Global oncology trends 2018. Innovation, expansion and disruption. 2018. Available at: https://www.iqvia.com/institute/reports/global-oncology-trends-2018. Accessed 28 June 2018.

28. Jit M, Brisson M, Portnoy A, Hutubessy R. Cost-effectiveness of female human papillomavirus vaccination in 179 countries: a PRIME modelling study. Lancet Glob Health. 2014;2(7):e406–14.

29. Lopes Gde L. Cost comparison and economic implications of commonly used originator and generic chemotherapy drugs in India. Ann Oncol. 2013;24(Suppl 5):v13–6.

30. Lopes Gde L Jr, de Souza JA, Barrios C. Access to cancer medications in low- and middle-income countries. Nat Rev Clin Oncol. 2013;10(6):314–22.

31. Machado K. Generic Herceptin approved in India. 2013. Available at: https://www.wsj.com/articles/generic-herceptin-approved-in-india-1385496898?tesla=y.

32. Mahal A, Karan A, Engelgau M. The economic implications of non-communicable disease for India. 2010. Available at: http://siteresources.worldbank.org/HEALTHNUTRITIONAND-POPULATION/Resources/281627-1095698140167/EconomicImplicationsofNCDforIndia.pdf.

33. Memorial Sloan Kettering Drug Pricing Lab. DrugAbacus. 2018. Available at: https://drug-pricinglab.org/tools/drug-abacus/. Accessed 28 June 2018.

34. Massard da Fonseca E, Bastos FI, Lopes G. Increasing access to oral anticancer medicines in middle-income countries: a case study of private health insurance coverage in Brazil. J Glob Oncol. 2016;2(1):39–46.

35. National Comprehensive Cancer Network. NCCN framework for resource stratification of NCCN guidelines. 2018. Available at: https://www.nccn.org/framework/default.aspx. Accessed 28 June 2018.

36. Perez EA, Romond EH, Suman VJ, Jeong JH, Sledge G, Geyer CE, Martino S, Rastogi P, Gralow J, Swain SM, Winer EP, Colon-Otero G, Davidson NE, Mamounas E, Zujewski JA, Wolmark N. Trastuzumab plus adjuvant chemotherapy for human epidermal growth factor receptor 2-positive breast cancer: planned joint analysis of overall survival from NSABP B-31 and NCCTG N9831. J Clin Oncol. 2014;32(33):3744–52.

37. Prager GW, Braga S, Bystricky B, Qvortrup C, Criscitiello C, Esin E, Sonke GS, Martínez GA, Frenel JS, Karamouzis M, Strijbos M, Yazici O, Bossi P, Banerjee S, Troiani T, Eniu A, Ciardiello F, Tabernero J, Zielinski CC, Casali PG, Cardoso F, Douillard JY, Jezdic S, McGregor K, Bricalli G, Vyas M, Ilbawi A. Global cancer control: responding to the growing burden, rising costs and inequalities in access. ESMO Open. 2018;3(2):e000285.

38. Prasad V. Do cancer drugs improve survival or quality of life? BMJ. 2017;359:j4528.

39. Prasad V, Mailankody S. Research and development spending to bring a single cancer drug to market and revenues after approval. JAMA Intern Med. 2017;177(11):1569–75.

40. Robertson J, Barr R, Shulman LN, Forte GB, Magrini N. Essential medicines for cancer: WHO recommendations and national priorities. Bull World Health Organ. 2016;94(10):735–42.

41. Rosenblatt E, Acuña O, Abdel-Wahab M. The challenge of global radiation therapy: an IAEA perspective. Int J Radiat Oncol Biol Phys. 2015;91(4):687–9.

42. Schnipper LE, Davidson NE, Wollins DS, Blayney DW, Dicker AP, Ganz PA, Hoverman JR, Langdon R, Lyman GH, Meropol NJ, Mulvey T, Newcomer L, Peppercorn J, Polite B, Raghavan D, Rossi G, Saltz L, Schrag D, Smith TJ, Yu PP, Hudis CA, Vose JM, Schilsky RL. Updating the American Society of Clinical Oncology value framework: revisions and reflections in response to comments received. J Clin Oncol. 2016;34(24):2925–34.

43. Shulman LN, Wagner CM, Barr R, Lopes G, Longo G, Robertson J, Forte G, Torode J, Magrini N. Proposing essential medicines to treat cancer: methodologies, processes, and outcomes. J Clin Oncol. 2016;34(1):69–75.
44. Strasser-Weippl K, Chavarri-Guerra Y, Villarreal-Garza C, Bychkovsky BL, Debiasi M, Liedke PE, Soto-Perez-de-Celis E, Dizon D, Cazap E, de Lima Lopes G, Touya D, Nunes JS, St Louis J, Vail C, Bukowski A, Ramos-Elias P, Unger-Saldaña K, Brandao DF, Ferreyra ME, Luciani S, Nogueira-Rodrigues A, de Carvalho Calabrich AF, Del Carmen MG, Rauh-Hain JA, Schmeler K, Sala R, Goss PE. Progress and remaining challenges for cancer control in Latin America and the Caribbean. Lancet Oncol. 2015;16(14):1405–38.
45. Szmulewitz RZ, Peer CJ, Ibraheem A, Martinez E, Kozloff MF, Carthon B, Harvey RD, Fishkin P, Yong WP, Chiong E, Nabhan C, Karrison T, Figg WD, Stadler WM, Ratain MJ. Prospective international randomized phase II study of low-dose abiraterone with food versus standard dose abiraterone in castration-resistant prostate cancer. J Clin Oncol. 2018;36(14):1389–95.
46. WHO. The selection and use of essential medicines. World Health Organ Tech Rep Ser. 2015;994:vii–xv, 1–546.
47. United Nations. Transforming our world: the 2030 agenda for sustainable development. 2018. Available at: https://sustainabledevelopment.un.org/post2015/transformingourworld. Accessed 28 June 2018.
48. U.S. Food and Drug Administration. Biosimilar product information. 2018. Available at: https://www.fda.gov/drugs/developmentapprovalprocess/howdrugsaredevelopedandapproved/approvalapplications/therapeuticbiologicapplications/biosimilars/ucm580432.htm. Accessed 28 June 2018.
49. Van Kriekinge G, Castellsagué X, Cibula D, Demarteau N. Estimation of the potential overall impact of human papillomavirus vaccination on cervical cancer cases and deaths. Vaccine. 2014;32(6):733–9.
50. Van Vlaenderen I, Canon JL, Cocquyt V, Jerusalem G, Machiels JP, Neven P, Nechelput M, Delabaye I, Gyldmark M, Annemans L. Trastuzumab treatment of early stage breast cancer is cost-effective from the perspective of the Belgian health care authorities. Acta Clin Belg. 2009;64(2):100–12.
51. Vergnenegre A, Massuti B, de Marinis F, Carcereny E, Felip E, Do P, Sanchez JM, Paz-Arez L, Chouaid C, Rosell R, Spanish Lung Cancer Group, Italian Association of Thoracic Oncology, French Lung Cancer Group. Economic analysis of first-line treatment with erlotinib in an EGFR-mutated population with advanced NSCLC. J Thorac Oncol. 2016;11(6):801–7.
52. Vergnenègre A, Chouaïd C. Review of economic analyses of treatment for non-small-cell lung cancer (NSCLC). Expert Rev Pharmacoecon Outcomes Res. 2018;18:519–28.
53. Wen F, Zheng H, Zhang P, Hutton D, Li Q. OPTIMAL and ENSURE trials-based combined cost-effectiveness analysis of erlotinib versus chemotherapy for the first-line treatment of Asian patients with non-squamous non-small-cell lung cancer. BMJ Open. 2018;8(4):e020128.
54. World Bank Open Data. Available at: https://data.worldbank.org/. Accessed 28 June 2018.
55. World Health Organization. The 2017 update, Global Health Workforce Statistics. Geneva. 2017. Available at: http://www.who.int/hrh/statistics/hwfstats/. Accessed 28 June 2018.
56. World Health Organization. Immunization, vaccines and biologicals. 2018. Available at: http://www.who.int/immunization/diseases/en/. Accessed 7 Sept 2018.
57. Young B, Surrusco M. Rx R&DMyths: the case against the drug industry's R&D "Scare Card." Washington, DC: Public Citizen's CongressWatch. 2001. Available at: https://www.citizen.org/sites/default/files/rdmyths.pdf. Accessed 8 July 2018.
58. Zubizarreta EH, Poitevin A, Levin CV. Overview of radiotherapy resources in Latin America: a survey by the International Atomic Energy Agency (IAEA). Radiother Oncol. 2004;73(1):97–100.
59. Zubizarreta E, Van Dyk J, Lievens Y. Analysis of global radiotherapy needs and costs by geographic region and income level. Clin Oncol (R Coll Radiol). 2017;29(2):84–92.

Chapter 7
Cancer Quackery and Fake News: Targeting the Most Vulnerable

David H. Gorski

Introduction

The following scenario is not hypothetical, but rather an amalgamation based on many cases that I have reviewed and discussed during the last 14 years that I have written about alternative cancer cures. It serves as a starting point to introduce and consider the forces that attract cancer patients and their families to cancer quackery and how in the right situation even seemingly obviously ridiculous forms of quackery can be sound attractive even to highly intelligent people.

Imagine that you are the parent of a young daughter. Imagine further that, after having developed normally and even hitting her developmental milestones earlier than average, your daughter starts to stumble and slur her speech. Naturally, as a parent, you become very concerned; so you take her to her pediatrician, who examines her, finds focal neurological signs, and orders an MRI of the brain. Terror seeps into your very being as you await the day of the test and, later, its results. Your fear goes nuclear as doctors tell you that your child has a diffuse intrinsic pontine glioma (DIPG), a highly aggressive cancer of the pons. It is inoperable, and oncologists tell you that, at best, palliative radiation therapy will delay the inevitable somewhat, meaning that your precious girl has a probable life expectancy of considerably less than a year. What do you do? If you are like most people, you would do what many, if not most, parents faced with this situation: Head straight to Google to find out if there are any promising treatments of which your child's oncologist might be unaware.

D. H. Gorski (✉)
Department of Surgery, Wayne State University School of Medicine and the Barbara Ann Karmanos Cancer Institute, Detroit, MI, USA
e-mail: gorskid@med.wayne.edu

© Springer Nature Switzerland AG 2019   95
E. H. Bernicker (ed.), *Cancer and Society*,
https://doi.org/10.1007/978-3-030-05855-5_7

Unfortunately, all too frequently, for many this search for information—and, above all, hope—leads cancer patients and families down a veritable rabbit hole of misinformation in the form of an ecosystem of websites, Twitter feeds, Facebook pages, weblogs, and YouTube channels promoting unproven and pseudoscientific treatments for cancer. These sites and channels are chock-full of glowing testimonials of patients who, if you believe their stories, were told to "go home and die" by their doctors but are now alive and well, often with no ill effects at all, thanks to the treatment(s), the site is promoting. These testimonials are often coupled with fake news and conspiracy theories about "big pharma," medicine, cancer, and even vaccines designed to sell "natural cures." Indeed, most of the social media sites promoting such "miracle cures," at least the ones that allow comments and/or contain discussion forums, form self-reinforcing echo chambers in which even mild and empathetic skepticism is attacked, leaving only true believers and potential converts, con artists, and their marks.

Most people instinctively understand the oft-repeated adage that if it sounds too good to be true, it almost certainly is. Sadly, all too often, staring into the approaching abyss of death or facing the realization that your child will soon no longer be with you can short-circuit even the staunchest skeptic's critical thinking skills. Let us now make this amalgamated scenario frighteningly concrete, to illustrate how purveyors of unproven treatments attract the desperate through a combination of distorted and even outright fake news and the multiple harms that use of these treatments can cause.

The Tragic Case of Amelia Saunders

In 2012, the parents of Amelia Saunders, a 3-year-old girl from Reading, England, faced the dilemma described above. In late 2011, Amelia's parents began noticing troubling symptoms, including difficulty with balance and a trembling left hand. Steady worsening of Amelia's symptoms, particularly her more frequent falls, led them to take her to her pediatrician, and on January 30, 2012, she was diagnosed with a large brain stem tumor [1]. Neurosurgeons attempted to remove the tumor but, because of its location and involvement of the brain stem, were unable to remove very much of the tumor mass. Unfortunately, the tissue that was recovered revealed grade 2 diffuse astrocytoma. As a result, the surgeons and oncologists were very honest and realistic with the family, telling them that Amelia probably only had a few months to live. They further explained that the survival benefit from radiation would most likely be measurable in weeks rather than months or years and that the side effects could be considerable.

Amelia's parents searched the Internet for alternatives, and their searches led them to websites promoting a Polish physician and expat in Houston named Stanislaw Burzynski. I have discussed Dr. Burzynski's history in great detail before [2], but for purposes of this chapter, a brief summary will suffice. First, Dr. Burzynski has never undertaken a fellowship in oncology. Second, in the mid-1970s while working as a junior researcher at the Baylor College of Medicine, he reported the discovery of endogenous peptides in human blood and urine that he believed to be part of the body's natural cancer suppression system that could "reprogram" cancer cells back to normal and dubbed them "antineoplastons" (ANPs) [3]. Ultimately they were characterized as mixtures of phenylacetic acid and phenylacetylglutamine, neither of which have shown much anticancer activity but which he learned to synthesize in his facility [4, 5].

Burzynski, however, became so convinced that he had made a major breakthrough in cancer treatment that, when he was unable to obtain approval for a clinical trial at Baylor, he left to start treating patients with his ANPs in his own private clinic, which later expanded to become the Burzynski Clinic. Over the course of the next four decades, he gained a reputation in alternative medicine circles as having a "cure" (or at least a treatment very much more effective than existing treatments) that was not only "natural" but had no side effects. That reputation was bolstered by media appearances, including on the *Sally Jessy Raphael Show* in the 1980s [6], as well as by a glowing chapter in a Suzanne Somers book [7], and promotion by websites and social media. A filmmaker named Eric Merola also released two long-form advertisements thinly disguised as documentaries, *Burzynski: Cancer Is A Serious Business* (2010) and *Burzynski: Cancer Is Serious Business, Part II* (2013).

Despite all this promotion and Burzynski's use of ANPs to treat patients for over 40 years, he has never published any compelling evidence supporting their efficacy [8], although in the 1990s, he did manage to set up a large number of clinical trials intended primarily as a means for him to administer ANPs [9]. Indeed, the existing clinical trials published by Burzynski are incomplete and unconvincing [10, 11], and he has been investigated by the FDA and prosecuted by the Texas Medical Board on multiple occasions [12]. Moreover, ANPs are toxic, the most common toxicity being hypernatremia, which has caused at least one child's death [13].

The Saunders family traveled to Houston to see Dr. Burzynski and began documenting her story on a website (ameliasmiracle.com) and a Facebook page of the same name. On February 28, 2012, the parents posted a video appeal, with the following message:

> Our daughter, Amelia, was diagnosed at the beginning of February with a very rare type of inoperable brain tumour. She has only a few months to live. We have a ray of hope – treatment for her is available at the Burzynski clinic in Houston, Texas. This treatment in total will cost around £200,000. We need to raise this money to allow Amelia to have the chance to live a normal life.

And raise money they did—prodigiously. Amelia's story first appeared in the press on March 8, 2012, and Eric Merola, the producer and director of the two Burzynski movies, interviewed the family, his plan being to feature her in the second film. By March 14 the family had raised £45,000, and by March 23 the family was on its way to Houston, having raised £75,000, where Amelia soon had a Hickman line inserted to receive ANPs. (Ultimately, the family would raise £245,000 in 12 weeks.) Amelia's case drew international attention, making her a minor celebrity. Sadly and not unexpectedly, though, by November 2012, Amelia was clearly getting worse, despite Burzynski's assurances that his ANPs were working [14]. Ultimately, the Saunders family decided to stop the ANPs, and Amelia died in hospice on January 6, 2013.

A Common Pattern

The case of Amelia Saunders was presented in such detail because it demonstrates a common pattern in the era of the web and social media by which the vulnerable are enticed into the hands of cancer quacks. Any of a number of others could have been chosen. While it is true that Stanislaw Burzynski is an unusual case, he is unusual mainly in that he has more of a veneer of science covering his pseudoscience than the average cancer quack. He has open clinical trials, a manufacturing facility to make his ANPs, and his own pharmacy. However, his business model is very similar to that of many cancer quacks in that he relies on a network of supportive websites and social media influencers to drive business to his clinic through a combination of glowing recommendations, claims of persecution by "big pharma" and the medical establishment, and even outright conspiracy mongering. The result is a combination of propaganda ranging from real news that are either very biased or in which claims made for Burzynski are not properly fact checked to outright fake news. Unsurprisingly, families who decide to pursue Burzynski's treatment also rely on these same networks. In Amelia Saunders' case, for instance, the British tabloid press aided and abetted Burzynski by facilitating fundraising for ANP treatment with poignant human interest stories, a pattern not unique to the UK.

It was not just the Saunders family, either. A large list of these patients can be found at The Other Burzynski Patient Group (theotherburzynskipatientgroup.wordpress.com), a weblog maintained by Robert Blaskiewicz dedicated to chronicling what is known about various patients who have been victimized by Burzynski. Sadly, even in 2018, Burzynski is still successfully recruiting patients using the same technique (Fig. 7.1).

Although Burzynski has been the focus as a prototypical example of how cancer quacks can leverage social media and traditional media, he is far from alone. For instance, the Hallwang Clinic in Germany, which promotes a mixture of conventional and alternative medicine plus experimental therapeutics administered outside the auspices of a clinical trial, has attracted patients from the UK, with much the same sorts of headlines and narratives about being a patient's "last chance"—along with, not surprisingly, similarly eye-popping price tags as Burzynski. For example, a UK woman named Pauline Gahan suffering from metastatic stomach cancer described to Emma Barnett on *5 Live Daily* in 2016 how she and her family had raised £300,000 by selling her house and car and renting the house back so that she could still live there. This paid for additional surgery and treatment of complications of a deep venous thrombosis, but it also paid for useless vitamin B infusions and a "liver detox" regimen, along with an unapproved veterinary drug. She also received whole-body hyperthermia and some very expensive immune checkpoint inhibitors.

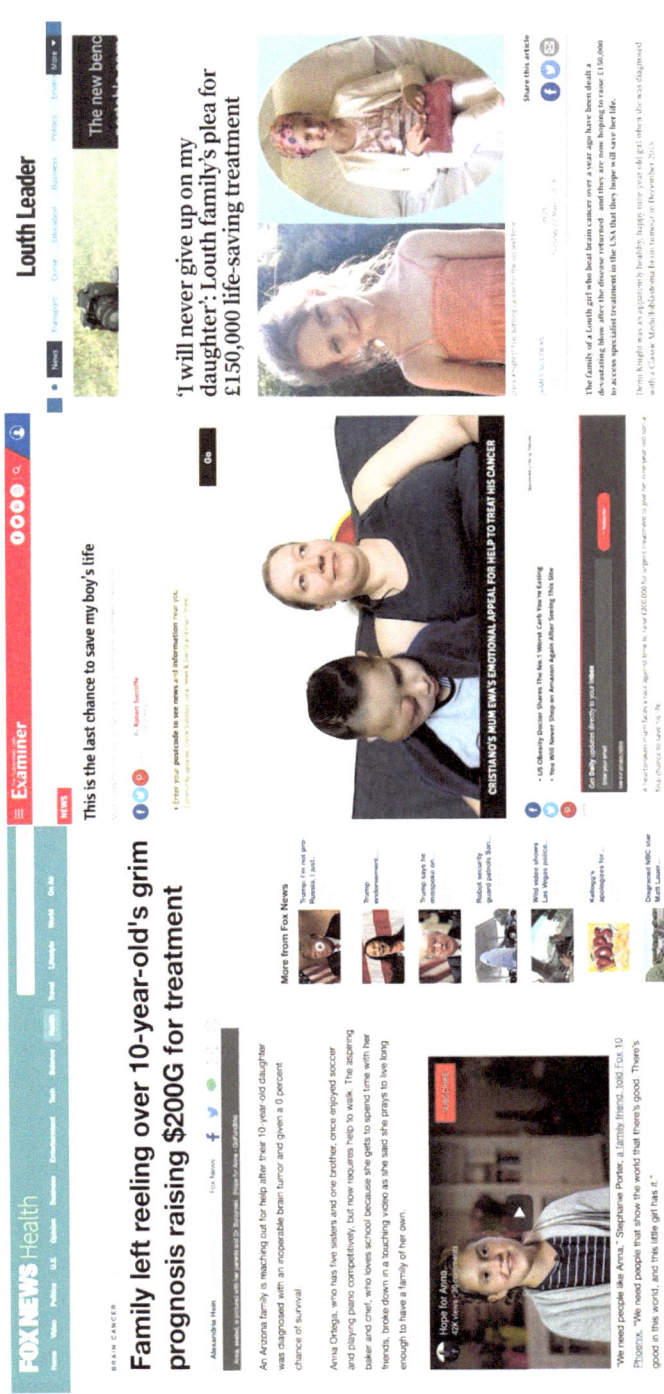

Fig. 7.1 Examples of media coverage of patients seeking care at the Burzynski Clinic. Note the narratives, including portraying Burzynski as the child's "last chance" and the need for large amounts of money. Left to right: Anna Ortega, Cristiano Sousa, and Anna Knight

According to its website (https://www.hallwang-clinic.com/your-oncological-jour-ney-cancer-treatment/advanced-treatment-concepts.html), Hallwang also offers many other unproven and pseudoscientific treatments, such as homeopathy, which has no scientific basis, naturopathy, dichloroacetate (an unproven experimental metabolic treatment), micronutrients and orthomolecular medicine, high-dose vitamin C, ozone therapy, hyperbaric oxygen, and "many more according to your needs." It is unclear how many of these other modalities Gahan availed herself of. Sadly, Gahan died in April 2017 [15]. She was not alone, either, in having been attracted to Hallwang. British actress Leah Bracknell was diagnosed with stage IV lung cancer in 2016 and also raised funds to go to Hallwang, £50,000 within 3 days, to receive a combination of "cutting-edge immunotherapy" and alternative medicine. As of March 2018, she was still alive but acknowledged that her treatment was "no longer working" [16].

There are many more examples of clinics selling proven combinations of experimental therapies and alternative medicine. For example, in Monterrey, Mexico, Dr. Alberto Siller and Alberto Garcia run *Instituto de Oncologia Intervencionista*, see pediatric DIPG patients at their *Clínica 0-19*, and treat them at a local hospital with a combination of "immunotherapy" and intra-arterial chemotherapy infusions into the brain stem. Not only have they never published their results, but they have refused to cooperate with the international oncological community to test their treatment. Indeed, their response to criticism about their refusal to publish details of their methods or their success rate for their invasive treatment is, quite literally, that they are "too busy treating…patients from around the world" to do so [17]. Yet they still charge patients from around the world, particularly the USA, the UK, and Australia, $11,000–30,000 per treatment, which can easily lead to charges of well in excess of $300,000. One family reported that the expense of treating their child had left the family "homeless, in debt and reliant on fundraising to keep up maintenance treatments" [17]. In 2018, an Australian girl named Annabelle Nguyen and her family were stranded in Mexico because Annabelle's tumor had recurred, putting her into a coma and leading to $2500 a day in medical expenses. Her family was unable to return to Australia because medical transport cost $250,000 [18]. She was not alone, either. A similar fate befell the family of a girl named Parker Monhollon.

There are far too many clinics like the Burzynski Clinic, Hallwang Clinic, or Clínica 0-19 to do a comprehensive review in this chapter, and that is without even considering the hundreds of "stem cell clinics" selling unproven stem cell therapies for everything from cancer to strokes, to heart disease, and to every chronic illness under the sun. However, common themes emerge from how such clinics are promoted around the world, to be discussed below. However, it needs to be pointed out that conventional media often aid and abet cancer quackery by emphasizing the human interest angle of stories of parents selling their homes, raising money using GoFundMe, and in general "overcoming all odds" to take their children with cancer to obtain "cutting-edge" or "experimental" treatments, rather than how such clinics are taking advantage of patients and parents. A recent example of this phenomenon is an incredibly poignant photo that went viral in June 2018. It portrayed a 6-year-

Fig. 7.2 Addy Joy Sooter's older brother Matthew comforts her hours before her death. This image went viral in June 2018, but none of the news stories that published this image described the treatment of Addy Joy's DIPG as anything other than "experimental therapy" in Monterrey or Mexico

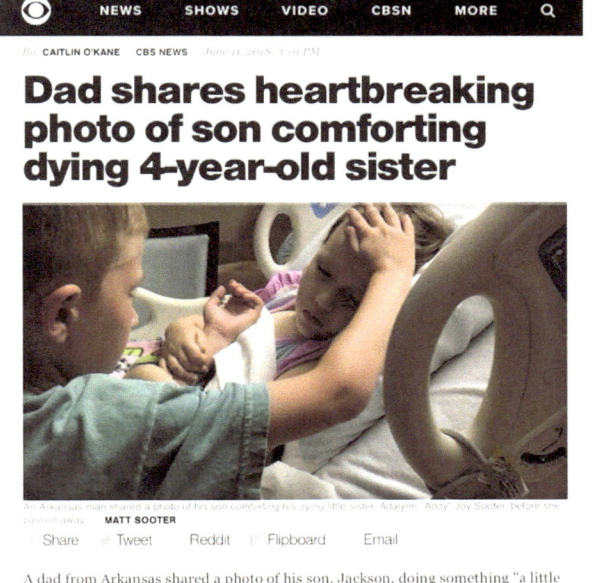

A dad from Arkansas shared a photo of his son, Jackson, doing something "a little boy should not have to." Jackson was comforting his 4-year-old sister, Addy, on her deathbed.

old boy named Jackson Sooter saying goodbye to his sister Addy Joy, who was dying of DIPG (Fig. 7.2). Notably missing, however, in news stories about the Sooters was any detail about her treatment or Clínica 0-19, where Addy Joy had been treated. In most news reports, the treatment was only described as an experimental treatment in Mexico.

The Messages of Cancer Quackery: Conspiracy, Anecdotes, and Fake News

Fake news has generally been defined as false or otherwise extremely exaggerated news stories used to generate money from ad revenue or to provoke a reaction, usually a negative one and often for political purposes. Unlike misinformation, bad reporting, or biased news, which is inaccurate because the reporter has confused, misreported, left out, or misinterpreted facts, fake news is created with the explicit intent to manipulate opinion and often reports incidents that never happened. By this definition, reporting by tabloids about cancer patients like Leah Bracknell or Amelia Saunders is not, strictly speaking, fake news, but rather biased news designed to attract readers and page clicks while, if one takes a charitable view of the reporters and editors publishing such stories, possibly accomplishing something good by helping the cancer patient. However, such stories, epitomized by reports in British tabloids like the *Daily Mail*, as well as appearing in tabloids, radio, and television reports around the world, do not help cancer patients. Quite the contrary, they are an integral part of the reason why quackery flourishes because they are basically toned-down versions of the messages found on cancer quackery websites and social media and thereby provide "respectable" mainstream versions of these messages.

But what are these messages, and how are they spread? In other words, how is cancer quackery sold? There are many strategies, but what follows are by far the most commonly used ones.

False Hope

Let us consider the introduction to this chapter again. If you are the parents of a child like Amelia Saunders, what do you want more than anything else? Obviously, any parent would want hope that what the physicians have told them is in error and hope that there is a way—any way—to save their child. Similarly, if you are an adult cancer patient, what you want more than anything else is hope that you can live a natural lifespan.

Just Google "cure cancer naturally" or "natural cancer cures" or something similar, and you will find a plethora of websites promising to be able to cure advanced cancers using "natural"—and, of course, nontoxic—treatments. You will find movies like *The Beautiful Truth: The World's Simplest Cure for Cancer*, which touts a treatment regimen concocted by Max Gerson, a German physician who immigrated to the USA in 1936 and claimed to have discovered a "dietary cure" for cancer. The Gerson protocol involves drinking freshly squeezed juices 10–13 times a day made from up to 20 lbs of fruit and vegetables, plus dozens of supplements a day, plus five coffee enemas a day [19]. Meat, milk, alcohol, canned or bottled foods, and tobacco were strictly prohibited. Although this protocol has never been shown to be effective against any cancer, it is quite popular in alternative cancer cure (ACC) circles, and Max Gerson's daughter Charlotte continued Gerson's quackery at a clinic in Tijuana—a haven for questionable cancer clinics for many years [20]—after his death. The clinic, now called the Northern Baja Gerson Center, is still in operation and charges $6250 a week (2 week minimum) for the protocol, plus "3 months' worth of supplements, 3–6 months of Coley's treatment, IV vitamin C, and pure, organic aloe vera, along with a myriad of other 'immuno-therapies' including various oxygen therapies" [http://www.gersontreatment.com/natural-cancer-treatment-2/].

Unfortunately, there is so much more. You will also find video series, such as Ty Bollinger's *The Truth About Cancer: A Global Quest*, which consists of nine episodes, ranging from an episode that uses deceptive arguments and cherry-picked studies to claim that conventional cancer treatment doesn't work to episodes touting cannabis, "advanced detoxing," "clean electricity," "superfoods," and juicing as cures for cancer. The series, unsurprisingly, concludes with an episode entitled *Cancer Conquerors & Their Powerful Stories of Victory*, which purports to show cancer patients "cured" by alternative treatments. (We will discuss such testimonials further below.) You will also encounter a video series like *Beyond Chemo: Outside the Box Cancer Therapies*, which is a six-episode series by naturopath Mark Stengler that touts basically the same treatments and claims as Bollinger's series and whose website (beyondchemo.org) greets visitors with the statement, "The $100 Billion Cancer Industry Will Do Anything to Keep these Safe, Natural Treatments from You!"

This brings us to the next method used to promote cancer quackery.

Conspiracy Theories

Common narratives found on websites and social media promoting quackery involve conspiracy theories. Indeed, it is arguable that the single most important factor making many of these quack cancer treatments seem plausible to the average person relates to conspiracy theories about cancer and cancer treatment. Alternative medicine is rife with these, particularly the belief that there are "natural cures" for cancer out there that "they" don't want you to know about (as in *Beyond Chemo*, above), the "they" being "big pharma," government (particularly the Food and Drug Administration), the medical industry, the American Medical Association, or a combination of these and others. One particularly outlandish conspiracy theory has been promoted by blogger Erin Elizabeth, who founded Health Nut News (healthnutnews.com) and lives with alternative medicine entrepreneur Dr. Joseph Mercola. The story, which began with the 2015 suicide of Dr. Jeff Bradstreet, an anti-vaccine icon who treated autism with an unproven remedy known as GcMAF, is that "holistic" doctors are being systematically murdered. As of June 2018, the death toll was said to have reached 86 [21], including Dr. Nicholas Gonzalez, who, prior to his death in 2015 from what appears to have been a heart attack, treated pancreatic cancer with a protocol very similar to the Gerson protocol that involved dietary interventions, supplements, oral pancreatic enzymes, and, of course, coffee enemas [22]. Unsurprisingly, part of the legend of Max Gerson includes the claims that he was "persecuted" for his "natural cure" and even that he was murdered.

Other conspiracy theories to be found on websites promoting cancer quackery often involve the claim either that "chemo doesn't work" or "chemo kills" but that big pharma and oncologists push it on hapless cancer patients in the service of big pharma's profits. Indeed, there is a claim that has been referred to as the "2% gambit," which claims that chemotherapy is only 2% effective. This claim is based primarily on one study that was notable for confusing curative chemotherapy with adjuvant chemotherapy [23]. It is not hard to find cartoons and illustrations on websites like NaturalNews.com portraying chemotherapy as deadly poison, cancer centers as Nazi death camps, and mammograms as a scam to create new cancer patients (www.naturalnews.com/CounterThink) or other conspiracies (Fig. 7.3).

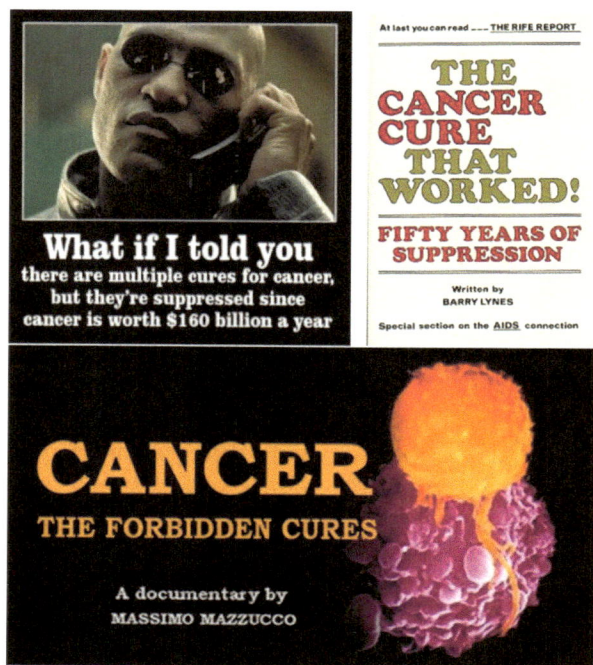

Fig. 7.3 Conspiracy theories in alternative medicine. Clockwise from upper right: (1) An Internet meme based on the popular science fiction movie The Matrix, variants of which are very common, some of which refer to the "red pill" from the movie that lets one see reality as it really is; (2) a book about the quack cancer device the Rife Frequency Instrument; (3) a documentary portraying "forbidden cures" for cancer, such as the Hoxsey therapy, as being suppressed. In all these narratives, there is a "conspiracy" by medical authorities, the government, and big pharma to "suppress natural cures"

Conspiracy theories in medicine are, unfortunately, understudied, but it is possible to glean some information. For example, in 2014, J. Eric Oliver reported a survey of 1351 adults and found that 63% of respondents had heard the claim that the FDA knew of "natural cures" for cancer but were keeping them from the public and 37% agreed that this claim was likely true [24]. An additional finding was that the number of conspiracy theories believed correlated with supplement use and negatively correlated with being vaccinated against influenza. Overall, half of all Americans believed at least one medical conspiracy theory, which suggests that such conspiracy theories have currency far outside of the quack fringe, and another study suggests that belief in conspiracy theories correlates with belief in political conspiracy theories [25]. Given the rise of fake news during the 2016 election, science-based physicians should expect that medical conspiracy theories are likely to become more prevalent as well, which will make persuading patients not to undertake treatments like Gerson's or Gonzalez's more difficult.

Testimonials

Cancer scientists and physicians have well-established standards of evidence required before a new cancer treatment is considered sufficiently effective and safe to be utilized:

1. Biological plausibility.
2. Preclinical data in cell culture and animal models suggesting efficacy.
3. Randomized clinical trials data showing efficacy against specific cancers either greater than placebo or efficacy noninferior to or greater than the existing standard of care in terms of overall survival. While it is true that science has become more accepting of surrogate endpoints (e.g., pathologic complete response, progression-free survival), the key point here is that there must be objective evidence of efficacy at a low enough cost in terms of toxicity to produce a favorable benefit-risk ratio.

Of course, oncologists and cancer scientists have to *learn* to think in terms of science and clinical trial data when assessing the efficacy of treatments. Such thinking does not come naturally to humans. What does come naturally to humans are stories, which is why one of the most powerful tools cancer quacks have is the alternative cancer cure (ACC) testimonial. Such testimonials feature a cancer patient who, according to the story, was cured by the treatment being promoted (or at least is doing *much* than his oncologists predicted). Such patients are often sympathetic, intelligent, and compelling storytellers, because the alternative medicine ecosystem's advertising system selects for such patients. Indeed, some of the most effective salespeople for ANPs were Burzynski patients featured in the movie and on a website The Burzynski Patient Group (burzynskipatientgroup.org).

It is very important when evaluating ACC testimonials to evaluate them for the following issues, beginning with the most common issue.

Conventional Therapy, Not the Alternative Medicine, Cured the Cancer

One of the most common forms of ACC testimonial is one I have sometimes referred to as the "skipped chemo" testimonial. Its power rests on the not knowing the difference between primary and adjuvant therapies. The basic form of such a testimonial is simple. A patient undergoes definitive surgery for a cancer treated primarily with surgery, decides not to undergo adjuvant therapy and instead chooses alternative medicine, and then attributes his or her survival to the alternative medicine, not the surgery. One example of this sort of testimonial is actress Suzanne Somers, who underwent breast-conserving surgery and sentinel lymph node biopsy for a hormone receptor-positive breast cancer in 2001 but then declined chemotherapy and tamoxifen in favor of Iscador, a mistletoe extract. She did accept radiation therapy, however, a decision she later wrote that she regretted [26]. Her story as described by her in her books and in the legend that has grown up around her is that she eschewed conventional chemotherapy in favor of alternative medicine and was cured of her cancer. A variant of this sort of ACC testimonial is a woman who claims to have had no surgery but in reality had undergone a surgical biopsy that had completely removed the tumor, i.e., the functional equivalent of a lumpectomy. Skin cancer diagnoses in which the lesion is removed by biopsy but further therapy is refused can also produce testimonials like this.

Another example of this sort of testimonial comes from a man named Chris Wark, who runs the Chris Beat Cancer website (chrisbeatcancer.com). In his testimonial, Wark states that at age 26 he was diagnosed with stage III colon cancer. The treatment for such a cancer is complete surgical excision of the segment of the colon containing the cancer with its associated mesentery, followed by chemotherapy. Wark, as is the case with all "skipped chemo" testimonials, admitted to undergoing definitive surgical resection of his cancer but refusing chemotherapy in favor of "nutrition and natural therapies to heal myself." I once ran an Adjuvant! Online (adjuvantonline.com) analysis of Wark's tumor based on his public descriptions of his disease and estimated that by refusing chemotherapy he had decreased his odds of surviving 5 years by 12–25%, depending on his stage and the chemotherapy regimen, but that he had started out with a 30–60% chance of survival with surgery alone. Unfortunately, nothing can convince Wark of this, and he has stated bluntly that surgery "does not cure cancer, especially not stage 3" [27]. He is, of course, incorrect. Since surviving cancer in 2003, Wark has gone on to run an Internet business as a "health and cancer coach" selling alternative medicine.

A variant of this sort of testimonial is one where a patient with a hematologic malignancy undergoes chemotherapy, stops after one or two cycles to pursue alternative medicine, and yet survives. In this case, again, conventional therapy has cured the cancer. The patient was simply fortunate enough that two cycles were enough and that he didn't require consolidation or maintenance chemotherapy. Unfortunately, such patients, like Alison Kelly, who developed locally advanced breast cancer and decided after surgery and part of her chemotherapy to stop all conventional therapy because of side effects, can end up in tabloids with headlines lauding her (Fig. 7.4).

Many of Burzynski's brain cancer patients' testimonials can be understood this way, because many of them undergo considerable conventional therapy with response before deciding to go the Burzynski clinic. In brain cancer, there is also a phenomenon known as pseudoprogression, in which edema from conventional chemotherapy and/or radiation therapy produces a "flare" on gadolinium-enhanced MRI that makes the tumor appear to be growing before it actually starts to shrink, and tumor necrosis can actually mimic tumor recurrence. As many as a third of brain cancer patients demonstrate this phenomenon during treatment [28]. More confoundingly, there is evidence that patients whose tumors demonstrate pseudoprogression during treatment might actually have better outcomes [29], thus selecting Burzynski's patients for better prognosis.

Fig. 7.4 Alison Kelly in the Irish newspaper *The Independent* on December 12, 2007. Newspapers frequently portray decisions to stop cancer treatment in a positive light, as brave, as "beating cancer my own way," in essence glorifying the choice of quackery over science-based medicine

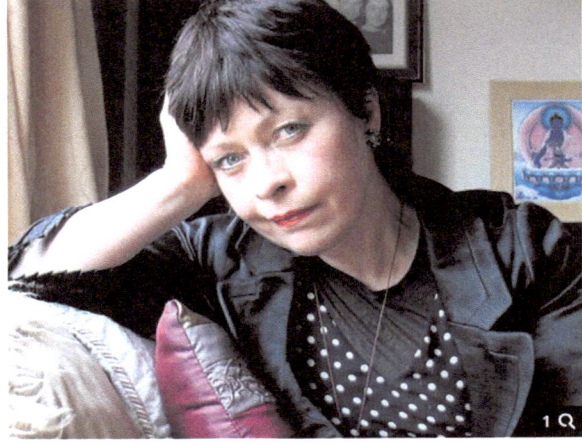

Lifestyle Health

I quit the cancer treatment and got better my own way

Picture of health: Alison Kelly says she has never felt healthier in her adult life after seemingly beating breast cancer on her own

Willie Dillon

Misread, Misunderstood, or Misrepresented Prognosis

One of the most common themes in alternative medicine cancer cure testimonials is that the "doctors sent me home to die." Oncologists and surgeons are, of course, obligated to be as honest as possible with their patients regarding the potential prognosis, but what patients frequently misunderstand (or doctors don't adequately communicate) is the inherent uncertainty in estimates of life expectancy after diagnosis. For many cancers, although the median survival might be relatively short, the "tale" on the survival curve can be fairly long, and outliers are more common than believed. For instance, from a historical study looking at data from decades ago [30], we know that the median survival of untreated breast cancer is approximately 2.7 years. However, at 7 years without treatment, 9% were still alive, and at 10 years, 3.6% were still alive. Alternative medicine cancer cure testimonials are particularly prone to survivorship bias, because it is only the survivors who live to produce testimonials.

Misdiagnosis

Finally, misdiagnosis is a surprisingly common reason explaining ACC testimonials. Again, Suzanne Somers provides an example in her book *Knockout* [26], in which she related an incident in which she was brought to the hospital for what sounded like an anaphylactic reaction. During her workup, she underwent CT scans, which showed what were presumed to be lung and liver masses. Of course, what a cancer patient who has undergone curative therapy most fears is recurrence of her cancer, and seeing such masses in a cancer patient always makes doctors think metastatic disease. The way that Somers told it, however, the hospital consulted an oncologist, who provided her with a grim prognosis, before it even had a tissue diagnosis, which actually turned out to be disseminated coccidioidomycosis. She was treated and recovered.

What to Look for in ACCs

Over the years, I have learned what to look for in ACC testimonials. The first thing I look for is whether the patient ever actually had cancer and, if so, exactly what type, plus all the relevant markers and prognostic factors. Not infrequently, this information is difficult or even impossible to discern, having been left out or obfuscated. Sometimes, however, it is laughably obvious that the patient giving the testimonial probably never had cancer. For example, I recently read *Heal Breast Cancer Naturally* by a chiropractor named Véronique Desaulniers-Chomniak [31]. In it Desaulniers-Chomniak describes "healing herself" of breast cancer. However, a skeptical reading of her anecdote easily reveals that there was never a proper tissue diagnosis. She had felt a lump and gone to an alternative medicine practitioner, who diagnosed her with breast cancer using "bioenergetic testing." The lump shrank. Of course, the most likely explanation is that she never had breast cancer in the first place. This particular form of misdiagnosis is particularly common among patients whose "diagnosis" is made by the alternative medicine practitioners using nonstandard diagnostic tests.

The Impact of Alternative Medicine on Cancer Patients

Thus far in this chapter, anecdotes have been presented to illustrate strikingly the deleterious effect of choosing alternative medicine rather than effective medicine on patients, but are there more objective data? Unfortunately, this is an area that is understudied. There are, however, studies that indicate that patients choosing alternative rather than science-based oncology to treat their cancers do themselves no favors.

The most recent of these studies was published in 2017 by Skyler Johnson and his colleagues at Yale University [32], in which the authors examined the correlation between alternative medicine use and cancer survival. They used data from the National Cancer Database, a clinical oncology database sourced from hospital registry data collected by the more than 1500 facilities accredited by the American

College of Surgeons Commission on Cancer (CoC). Its data cover more than 70% of newly diagnosed cancer cases nationwide and are used to develop quality improvement initiatives and set quality standards for cancer care in many hospitals across the USA. Identifying patients who underwent alternative medical treatment of cancer by those coded as "other-unproven: cancer treatments administered by nonmedical personnel" and who also did not receive CCT, defined as chemotherapy, radiotherapy, surgery, and/or hormone therapy, Skyler et al. examined correlation between survival and alternative medicine use as the primary treatment. Patients with metastatic disease at diagnosis, stage IV disease based on the American Joint Committee on Cancer (AJCC) staging system, receipt of upfront treatment with palliative intent, and unknown treatment status or clinical or demographic characteristics were excluded, leaving 280 patients to compare to those receiving standard care.

The authors identified only 280 patients who fit their criteria and noted that patients in the alternative medicine group were likely to be younger, female, and have a lower Charlson-Deyo Comorbidity Score (CDCS). In multivariate analyses controlling for clinical and demographic factors, the authors found that patients undergoing alternative cancer treatments were more likely to have breast cancer and higher education, Intermountain West or Pacific regions of residence, stage 2 or 3 disease, and a lower CDCS, consistent with the conclusion that patients who choose alternative cancer cures tend to be of higher socioeconomic status and education, as well as healthier than average. They were also more likely to have stage 2 or 3 disease. Survival statistics for four cancers (breast, prostate, lung, and colorectal) were analyzed. Unsurprisingly, the risk of death was higher for three out of the four cancers examined. Specifically, the hazard ratio (HR) for death was 2.5 (95% confidence interval [CI] 1.88–3.27); 5.68 for breast cancer (CI 3.22–10.04); 2.17 for lung cancer (CI 1.42–3.32); and 4.57 for colorectal cancer (CI 1.66–12.61). The difference observed was not significant for prostate cancer, likely because the survival with conventional therapy was so high to begin with. Also, prostate cancer tends to have a long natural course, and in this study, the numbers were small.

There are other studies showing an adverse effect. In 2006, Chang et al. carried out a chart review [33] of patients in their community practice who refused or delayed recommended treatment of their breast cancer to pursue alternative therapies, dividing them into groups as follows: patients who refused surgical treatment altogether; patients who delayed appropriate surgical treatment to pursue alternative treatments; patients who refused adequate sampling of the lymph nodes; patients who refused procedures to ensure adequate local control (additional surgery and/or radiation therapy); and patients who refused chemotherapy. Survival was compared to that expected in patients with disease of the same type and stage. Of patients who refused surgery, none of the six patients identified were stage IV (metastatic disease) at initial diagnosis. However, five out of these six patients who returned to the surgeons doing the study had progressed to stage IV, with a median time of follow-up of 14 months, with one death within a year. There were also five patients identified who initially refused surgery in favor of alternative medicine, all of whom were stage II or III. The median time between diagnosis and surgery was 37 months. All five demonstrated progression of their disease, with three progressing to stage IV disease and one of these dying of metastatic disease. Thus, 10/11 patients who refused surgery experienced significant disease progression, with 8/11 of these progressing to stage IV disease and 2/11 dying within the short time frame of the study.

A follow-up study from the same practice 5 years later [34] showed results as grim. In the group that refused surgery, 96.2% of patients experienced progression of their cancer, and 50% died of their disease. The mean stage at diagnosis in this group was II, but the mean stage when patients in this group re-presented after primary treatment with alternative medicine was IV. In the group refusing adjuvant therapy, progression occurred in 86.2% of those in the ASG, and 20% died of disease. Overall, in the surgery group, the expected mean 10-year survival calculated for those omitting surgery was 69.5%. In comparison the actual observed 10-year survival for these patients was 36.4% at a median follow-up of 33 months. For the patients who delayed surgery to undertake alternative treatments, the figures were 73.6% expected survival versus a 60% observed survival. The harm caused by declining conventional treatment in favor of alternative medicine is supported by another study [35] of 185 women in the Northern Alberta Health Region who declined recommended primary standard treatments, resulting in a median delay in instituting effective treatment of up to 101 months. The 5-year overall survival rates were 43.2% for those who refused standard treatments and 81.9% for those who received them, and disease-specific survival were 46.2% vs. 84.7%. Finally, even in patients who undergo conventional therapy, the use of certain "complementary and alternative medicine" (CAM) modalities is associated with delays in diagnosis and treatment [36] and delays in chemotherapy [37].

Conclusions

The use of alternative medicine in place of known effective cancer therapy remains a major problem and threat to the treatment of cancer patients, and use of such treatments has been linked conclusively to much poorer outcomes. Unproven, ineffective, and potentially harmful therapies are promoted primarily through an ecosystem of websites, YouTube videos, documentaries, and social media groups on Facebook and Twitter devoted to promoting "natural" treatments through a combination of fake news, false hope, conspiracy theories about oncology, and alternative cancer cure testimonials, whose messages sometimes unfortunately bleed over into conventional media through human interest stories of cancer patients seeking treatment at alternative medicine clinics. Oncologists and others taking care of cancer patients need to be aware of the scope of the problem, the fallacies in the messages used to promote quackery, and how to treat patients nonjudgmentally if they are to minimize the impact of these harmful messages.

References

1. Blaskiewicz R. Burzynski patient Amelia S.'s story [Weblog]. 2014 [cited June 2, 2018]. Available from: https://theotherburzynskipatientgroup.wordpress.com/2013/06/03/burzynski-patient-amelia-s-s-story/.
2. Gorski DH. Stanislaw Burzynski: four decades of an unproven cancer cure. Skept Inq. 2014;38(2):36–43.
3. Burzynski SR. Antineoplastons: biochemical defense against cancer. Physiol Chem Phys. 1976;8(3):275–9.
4. Green S. 'Antineoplastons'. An unproved cancer therapy. JAMA. 1992;267(21):2924–8.
5. Green S. Stanislaw Burzynski and "antineoplastons" [Internet]. 2001 [cited June 26, 2018]. Available from: http://www.quackwatch.org/01QuackeryRelatedTopics/Cancer/burzynski1.html.
6. Barrett S. Questionable cancer therapies [Internet]. 2002 [cited June 5, 2018]. Available from: http://www.quackwatch.org/01QuackeryRelatedTopics/Cancer/burzynski1.html.
7. Somers S. Dr. Stanislaw Burzynski. Knockout: interviews with doctors who are curing cancer and how to prevent getting it in the first place. New York: Crown Publishing; 2009. p. 59–86.
8. The antineoplaston anomaly: how a drug was used for decades in thousands of patients, with no safety, efficacy data. Cancer Lett. 1998;24(36):1.
9. Jaffe RA. The Burzynski Wars. Galileo's lawyer: courtroom battles in alternative health, complementary medicine, and experimental treatments. Houston: Thumbs UP Press; 2008. p. 37–134.
10. Burzynski SR, Janicki TJ, Burzynski GS, Marszalek A. The response and survival of children with recurrent diffuse intrinsic pontine glioma based on phase II study of antineoplastons A10 and AS2-1 in patients with brainstem glioma. Childs Nerv Syst. 2014;30:2051–61. Epub 2014/04/11.
11. Ogata Y, Matono K, Tsuda H, Ushijima M, Uchida S, Akagi Y, et al. Randomized phase II study of 5-fluorouracil hepatic arterial infusion with or without antineoplastons as an adjuvant therapy after hepatectomy for liver metastases from colorectal cancer. PLoS One. 2015;10(3):e0120064. Epub 2015/03/20.
12. Figg WD. Antineoplastons: when is enough enough? Lancet Oncol. 2018;19(6):733–4. Epub 2018/06/13.
13. Szabo L. Doctor accused of selling false hope to families. USA Today. 2013. Available from: https://www.usatoday.com/story/news/nation/2013/11/15/stanislaw-burzynski-cancer-controversy/2994561/.
14. Blaskiewicz R. Skeptic activists fighting for Burzynski's cancer patients. Skept Inq. 2014;38(2):43–8.
15. Gellman L. The last resort [Internet]. 2018 [cited May 25, 2018]. Available from: https://longreads.com/2018/03/22/the-last-resort/.
16. Brennan S. Terminally ill Emmerdale star Leah Bracknell reveals how she struggles to stay positive as she faces leaving her two daughters behind as she reaches her 'sell-by date'. Daily Mail. 2018. Available from: http://www.dailymail.co.uk/femail/article-5467747/Terminally-ill-Leah-Bracknell-reveals-fear-leaving-daughters.html.
17. Hansen J. Secretive Mexican brain cancer clinic to be investigated by Australian expert. The Daily Telegraph. 2018. Available from: https://www.dailytelegraph.com.au/news/nsw/secretive-mexican-brain-cancer-clinic-to-be-investigated-by-australian-expert/news-story/746147a2222d50d86c9b0927fcb9b840.
18. Parents' desperate quest to bring Perth brain tumour sufferer Annabelle Nguyen home from Mexico. The West Australian. 2018. Available from: https://thewest.com.au/news/perth/parents-desperate-quest-to-bring-perth-brain-tumour-sufferer-annabelle-nguyen-home-from-mexico-ng-b88875738z.
19. Unproven methods of cancer management: Gerson method. CA Cancer J Clin. 1990;40(4):252–6.

20. Questionable cancer practices in Tijuana and other Mexican border clinics. CA Cancer J Clin. 1991;41(5):310–9.
21. Elizabeth E. 86th doctor found dead in GA river, CDC & Atlanta PD give conflicting stories [Internet]. 2018 [cited July 1, 2018]. Available from: https://www.healthnutnews. com/86th-doctor-found-dead-in-ga-river-cdc-atlanta-pd-give-conflicting-stories/.
22. Chabot JA, Tsai WY, Fine RL, Chen C, Kumah CK, Antman KA, et al. Pancreatic proteolytic enzyme therapy compared with gemcitabine-based chemotherapy for the treatment of pancreatic cancer. J Clin Oncol. 2010;28(12):2058–63. Epub 2009/08/19.
23. Morgan G, Ward R, Barton M. The contribution of cytotoxic chemotherapy to 5-year survival in adult malignancies. Clin Oncol (R Coll Radiol). 2004;16(8):549–60. Epub 2005/01/06.
24. Oliver JE, Wood T. Medical conspiracy theories and health behaviors in the United States. JAMA Intern Med. 2014;174(5):817–8. Epub 2014/03/19.
25. Galliford N, Furnham A. Individual difference factors and beliefs in medical and political conspiracy theories. Scand J Psychol. 2017;58(5):422–8. Epub 2017/08/08
26. Somers SA. Cancer story—mine. Knockout: interviews with doctors who are curing cancer and how to prevent getting it in the first place. New York: Crown Publishing; 2009. p. 3–17.
27. Walia A. Man with stage 3 colon cancer refuses chemotherapy & treats himself with vegan diet [Weblog]. 2013 [cited June 3, 2018]. Available from: https://www.collective-evolution. com/2013/07/21/man-with-stage-3-colon-cancer-refuses-chemotherapy-cures-himself-with-vegan-diet/.
28. Fink J, Born D, Chamberlain MC. Pseudoprogression: relevance with respect to treatment of high-grade gliomas. Curr Treat Options in Oncol. 2011;12(3):240–52.
29. Sanghera P, Perry J, Sahgal A, Symons S, Aviv R, Morrison M, et al. Pseudoprogression following chemoradiotherapy for glioblastoma multiforme. Can J Neurol Sciences Le journal canadien des sciences neurologiques. 2010;37(1):36–42.
30. Bloom HJ. The natural history of untreated breast cancer. Ann N Y Acad Sci. 1964;114(2):747–54.
31. Desaulniers-Chomniak V. Healing breast cancer naturally: 7 essential steps to beating breast cancer. TKC Publishing, Incs; 2016. p. 162.
32. Johnson SB, Park HS, Gross CP, Yu JB. Use of alternative medicine for cancer and its impact on survival. J Natl Cancer Inst. 2018;110(1):121–4. Epub 2017/09/20.
33. Chang EY, Glissmeyer M, Tonnes S, Hudson T, Johnson N. Outcomes of breast cancer in patients who use alternative therapies as primary treatment. Am J Surg. 2006;192(4):471–3. Epub 2006/09/19.
34. Han E, Johnson N, DelaMelena T, Glissmeyer M, Steinbock K. Alternative therapy used as primary treatment for breast cancer negatively impacts outcomes. Ann Surg Oncol. 2011;18(4):912–6. Epub 2011/01/13.
35. Joseph K, Vrouwe S, Kamruzzaman A, Balbaid A, Fenton D, Berendt R, et al. Outcome analysis of breast cancer patients who declined evidence-based treatment. World J Surg Oncol. 2012;10:118. Epub 2012/06/28.
36. Mohd Mujar NM, Dahlui M, Emran NA, Abdul Hadi I, Wai YY, Arulanantham S, et al. Complementary and alternative medicine (CAM) use and delays in presentation and diagnosis of breast cancer patients in public hospitals in Malaysia. PLoS One. 2017;12(4):e0176394. Epub 2017/04/28.
37. Greenlee H, Neugut AI, Falci L, Hillyer GC, Buono D, Mandelblatt JS, et al. Association between complementary and alternative medicine use and breast cancer chemotherapy initiation: the Breast Cancer Quality of Care (BQUAL) Study. JAMA Oncol. 2016;2(9):1170–6. Epub 2016/06/01.

Chapter 8
The Adoption of Artificial Intelligence in Cancer Pathology and Imaging

Stephen T. C. Wong

Staying ahead in the fast-tracking artificial intelligence (AI) race today requires good understanding of the technology and products by physicians and executives to make informed decisions about when, where, and how to employ AI in their clinical practice. But what is artificial intelligence? Generally speaking, it is referred to as the study of constructing and/or programming learning computers or machines imbued with human-like characteristics that can be utilized to make decisions in a specific case in the service of a specified goal. Well-known examples include proving a mathematical theorem, performing a medical diagnosis, interpreting legal advice, playing a complex game of Go or chess, or navigating and driving an autonomous vehicle. Often these tools outperform human beings at a given task. This type of artificial intelligence, also known as narrow or weak AI, which is focused on one specific task, is defined in contrast to strong AI that refers to a computer or a machine with commonsense, consciousness, sentience, and mind or with the ability to apply intelligence to any problem, rather than just one specific problem [1, 2]. Weak AI, in contrast to strong AI, does not attempt to perform the full range of human cognitive abilities. All currently existing systems considered artificial intelligence of any sort are weak AI at most.

Around three-quarters of a century ago, Walter Pitts, Alan Turing, Stephen Kleene, and Warren McCulloch defined the two schools of thought on AI that form the theoretical foundation and philosophical division. In 1943, Warren McCulloch, a neuroscientist, and Walter Pitts, a logician, produced their groundbreaking work on finite-state machines as a model of computation and launched the field of artificial neural networks [3]. Meanwhile, in 1950, Alan Turing published a seminal paper focused on logic inferences [4]. Then, in December of 1951, Stephen Kleene

S. T. C. Wong (✉)
Systems Medicine and Bioengineering Department, Houston Methodist Cancer Center and Houston Methodist Research Institute, Houston, TX, USA
e-mail: stwong@houstonmethodist.org

© Springer Nature Switzerland AG 2019

E. H. Bernicker (ed.), *Cancer and Society*,
https://doi.org/10.1007/978-3-030-05855-5_8

further clarified the work of McCulloch and Pitts in a project funded by RAND research with a memorandum that was formally published in 1956 [5]. In the same year, John McCarthy formally coined the term "artificial intelligence" during the 1956 workshop of the Dartmouth Summer Research Project on AI [6, 7], at which he primarily referred to AI as logic inference or symbolic processing, as opposed to neural networks, which were defined by McCulloch and Pitts and refined by Kleene.

From that period through the 2000s, the AI field has experienced several buildup cycles and winters, based on a number of challenges, followed by disappointment and criticism, followed by research funding cuts, and followed by renewed interest years or decades later. An AI winter refers to a period of reduced funding and interest in artificial intelligence research and was coined by analogy to the idea of a nuclear winter. The surge of interest in AI and its resounding success since the 2010s are due to advances related to neural networks school of AI—in particular, machine learning and deep learning—not in the logic inference school of AI, though both are complementary. Suffice to say, the field of AI has evolved through cycles of obscurity, conceptualization, enthusiasm and optimism, and failure and disappointment. Now, many AI applications are embedded in the infrastructure of various industries [8, 9].

The healthcare industry has noticed of the surge and potential of AI. However, as AI implementation strategies and applications are being developed, it is becoming increasingly clear that incorporating AI into healthcare will inevitably be overwrought with a variety of complications. AI is the road that leads to the way of the future, though it may not be as revolutionary as portrayed by the media: AI as androids that emulate complex human emotions—as demonstrated by the fictional android superhero, Vision, from Marvel's *The Avengers*, or C-3P0 from the motion picture *Star Wars*, or harbingers of destruction as AI evolves beyond or maliciously complies with human programming directives, as seen in the HAL 9000 computer from the novel *2001: A Space Odyssey*. Many qualms stem from the idea that advancements in AI will bring to that point in history when AI surpasses human intelligence, leading to an unimaginable revolution in human affairs. Or, they wonder whether artificial intelligence will control us, turning us, in effect, into cyborgs instead. Though such ideas are interesting issues to contemplate and debate, they are not imperative. Interestingly, although it has been reported that AI systems have eclipsed clinicians in detecting and diagnosing specific diseases [10–12], AI is not a universal panacea poised to supersede the medical profession any time in the near future; rather, over time AI will transform the practice of medicine by enhancing the physician's efficiency and accuracy, supplementing the value of care given to patients.

Recent growing interest in incorporating AI into a number of industries can be attributed to the rise of deep learning [13], a process through which AI recognizes patterns using various forms of neural networks based on the availability of big data repositories and inexpensive and easy access to computational processing power and sometimes by means of rapid data acquisition via digital camera, imaging scanners, electronic appliances, remote sensors, or the Internet of Things (IoT) [14]. When applied to medicine, deep learning applications can be trained with large amounts of annotated datasets, thereby freeing medical specialists to focus on more productive tasks and projects. The potential of AI is limitless and can serve as a great boon in improving healthcare delivery in clinical practice [15]. In particular, deep learning, or broader machine learning, type of AI is making inroads in clinical research and practices, including oncology and notably, medical imaging specialties such as radiology of relevance to precision oncology. Radiologists have experimented with AI automation to improve accuracy with regard to diagnostic imaging. Due to the direct acquisition of patient images in digital form for central archival and softcopy review, the radiology practice readily incorporates AI into the clinical environment. An established digital imaging infrastructure, such as picture archiving and communication systems (PACS), allows AI to be seamlessly embedded into radiology workflow, thus facilitating the translation and transmission of large quantities of data within minutes. For patient images generated by different imaging modalities (e.g., positron emission tomography (PET), magnetic resonance imaging (MRI), computed tomography (CT), X-ray, mammograms, and ultrasound), deep learning AI can potentially be automated to pinpoint areas of interest and diagnosis or even check the quality of diagnostic or claim reports by payers or other care providers.

This is evidenced by the large number of scientific presentations, lectures, and vendor product offerings at recent radiology and healthcare information technology conferences on AI applications in medical imaging. During 2017 and the upcoming 2018 HIMSS conferences, leading health tech companies, such as IBM, Philips, GE, Agfa, Microsoft, and Siemens, have already started integrating AI into their medical imaging software systems. GE demonstrated AI software to predict the operational impact on imaging departments when a person declares sickness or if patient volumes increase. Philips Healthcare's Illumeo software incorporated adaptive intelligent algorithms to pull in related prior radiology exams automatically. The user can select an area of the anatomy in a specific image view, and the embedded AI algorithm will find and open prior imaging studies to display and compare. In the case for cancer diagnostic imaging, just with a couple clicks to focus on the tumor in the image, the AI program will automatically quantitate the image and then perform the same measures on the priors, presenting a side-by-side comparison of the tumor assessment. Such AI tools would reduce the time involved with tumor tracking assessment and, therefore, accelerate clinical workflow. Microsoft launched Healthcare NExT, a new initiative that attempts to bring together artificial intelligence, health research, and the expertise of industry partners aiming to improve quality of life of patients and manage diseases. In addition, the vast commercial potential of AI in disease management has attracted significant venture capital investments, and healthcare has consistently been the top industry for AI deals in recent years [16]. Several companies and startups have recently been formed in the field, showing prototype software that applies AI to sift through massive amounts of big image data or offer immediate clinical decision support for appropriate use criteria, the optimal test or imaging procedures to make a diagnosis or offer differential diagnoses.

Agfa's AI application exemplifies how the technology works. A digital radiography (DR) chest X-ray exam is pulled out, and IBM's Watson computer system reviewed the image and determined that the patient had small-cell lung cancer and evidence of both lung and heart surgery [17]. Watson then searched the PACS, EMR (electronic medical record), and departmental reporting systems to bring in prior chest imaging studies; cardiology report information; medications the patient is taking; patient history relevant to them having chronic obstructive pulmonary disease (COPD) and a history of smoking that might relate to their current exam; recent lab reports; oncology patient encounters including chemotherapy; and radiation therapy treatments. When the radiologist opens the study, all this information is presented in a coherent format and greatly enhances the picture of this patient's health and thus improves the radiologist's understanding of the patient to improve the diagnosis, therapies, and resulting patient outcomes without adding more burden on the clinicians. This application exemplifies IBM's Watson Imaging solutions that aim to analyze both structured and unstructured patient, population, and medical research data residing within disconnected silos in a health system. It strives to organize and present available information in a probability-driven manner in order to assist clinicians and caregivers in making objective decisions, whether at a reading workstation or at the point of care. However, it is worth noting that for such AI technology to function, a significant amount of systems integration work of underlying clinical databases of the healthcare provider institution, e.g., PACS, EMR, and departmental reporting information systems, must be performed to feed into IBM's Watson, and often careful validation of the quality of integrated data is required. This adds considerable costs and time effort in clinical implementation; a Watson Health project typically runs over a few to tens of millions and thus faces challenges in the readiness of local institutions' information infrastructure for integration and the justification of return of investments to hospital administration. This may contribute to the slow adoption of Watson by healthcare providers.

The earlier is cancer detection, the easier it is to treat the disease. But too often, cancers are diagnosed at a late stage when they are much more difficult to treat. The use of AI such as machine and deep learning to interrogate medical and nonmedical datasets is a promising strategy for early detection of cancer. Access to vast quantities of patient data and images is needed to feed the AI software algorithms educational materials to learn from. Sorting through massive amounts of big data is a major component of how AI learns what is important for clinicians and what data elements are related to various disease states and gains clinical understanding. It is a similar process to medical students learning their field, but much more educational input than what is comprehensible by humans can be learned. The first step in machine learning software is for it to ingest medical textbooks and care guidelines and then review examples of clinical cases. Unlike human students, the number of cases AI has access to and can learn numbers in the millions.

For cases where the AI did not accurately determine the disease state or found incorrect or irrelevant data, software programmers go back and refine the AI algorithm iteration after iteration until the AI software gets it right in the majority of cases. In cancer, there are plethora of variables that makes it difficult to always arrive at the correct diagnosis for people or machines. However, percentage wise, experts now say AI software reading medical imaging studies can often match or, in some cases, outperform human radiologists, especially in cases of rare diseases or presentations, whereas a radiologist might only see a handful of such cases during their entire career. AI has the advantage of reviewing hundreds or even thousands of these rare studies from archives to become proficient at reading them and identify a proper diagnosis. Also, unlike the human mind, the data can be extracted exactly as the original, presenting itself as fresh evidence each iteration.

AI algorithms read medical images similar to radiologists, by identifying patterns. AI systems are trained using vast numbers of exams to determine what normal anatomy looks like on scans from CT, MRI, or ultrasound. Then, abnormal cases are used to train the eye of the AI system to identify anomalies, similar to computer-aided detection (CAD) software. However, unlike CAD, which just highlights areas a radiologist may want to take a closer look at, AI software has a more analytical cognitive ability based on much more clinical data and reading experience than previous generations of CAD software. Experts who are helping develop AI for medical imaging often refer to the cognitive ability as "CAD that works."

Surging interest and active investment of AI in radiology have inspired pathologists to incorporate AI into their practices as well. However, with a few applications of surgical pathologic diagnosis of tumors, such as IBD (inflammatory bowel disease) diagnosis in gastrointestinal (GI) biopsies or the diagnosis of nephropathies, currently it is difficult to envision how AI can be integrated effectively into routine pathology practice, as a digital workflow platform for surgical pathology does not yet exist—a barrier that has to be dealt with and, in surgical pathology subspecialties, image analysis from the tissue slide has to be combined with clinical data and observations in a large percentage of cases to arrive at diagnosis—pathologic image alone does not get one there in these "medical" forms of surgical pathology.

Pathology departments generate high-resolution microscopy images that, unlike their counterparts in radiology, do not correlate to equivalent standardized digital imaging formats and workflow. Furthermore, images in pathology require a manual process of tissue biopsy, specimen preparation, and staining before digitization. Even assuming high-speed AI algorithms can be developed to accurately detect and diagnose digitized pathologic images, the productivity gain of automation would be rather minimal [15]. Direct acquisition of pathologic images with digital modalities such as bright-field and whole slide fluorescence scanning is extremely rare in current pathology practice. There are research projects on digitized pathologic images for telepathology. One system that assists in the digitization of pathologic images is whole slide imaging (WSI), which involves scanning the whole tissue on glass slides and digitizing the images. With WSI, many pathology slides can be analyzed efficiently within a relatively short period; nevertheless, the system suffers from complications associated with acceptance, speed, the inability to digitize all types of tissues, and data resolution, storage, and regulation [18]. In September of 2017, the Food and Drug Administration approved the first WSI system [19], which may encourage the pathology community to begin standardizing and digitizing on a larger scale, streamlining the exchange of information.

Furthermore, the multidimensional nature of radiologic images allows imaging specialists to view them on a 2D, 3D, or 4D plane, which delivers rich information for AI pattern recognition. Conversely, pathologic images are normally digitized for

2D presentation, which does not provide as much information on the sample as it would on a 3D or 4D plane. The fact that there is no established, standardized digital pathologic imaging workflow complicates the exchange and translation of information to other information systems, physicians, and health systems [20]. The lack of accessibility to large centralized image archives of digitized pathologic images, compared to medical imaging archives such as picture archiving and communication systems (PACS), creates additional hurdles to successfully integrating AI into the pathology practice. The implementation of such an image data warehouse requires an immense capital investment for storage and administration that may not be feasible or necessary for smaller clinics and hospitals. Pathologic imaging management in the cloud computing environment may be a viable solution if there are adequate security and privacy issue safeguards and the speed of image transfer over the Internet is sufficient. Should a standardized digital imaging infrastructure be established in pathology, it will pave the way for AI to become a powerful asset for pathologists who seek to better bridge the gap between clinical research and patient care.

Complicating matters further is the fact that applying deep learning or other AI tools in medical diagnosis requires a multimodality approach in which data from patient images, as well as demographic information, medical history, and other laboratory and clinical results, are extracted and compiled to integrate into decision-making or risk assessment models. Nonetheless, even with the recent widespread implementation of electronic health records in the United States, as it stands today, a significant amount of clinical data remains in unstructured free-text reports that are challenging to extract efficiently—even with NLP (natural language processing) tools, another AI technique. Often there is no unanimous or standard form of electronic documentation; therefore, investing in translational tools is essential. But with each additional AI tool and human resource invested in processing and mining those systems, net efficiency gains and the effectiveness of AI integrated into clinical practice face diminishing returns.

There are several other barriers of entry for AI become more commonplace in medicine, including imaging specialties like radiology and pathology. One unresolved issue is where legal responsibility lies, e.g., who is accountable for an action resulting from an AI-based decision. Legal representation in the medical field is a significant barrier in the process of implementing new procedures, pharmaceuticals, and technologies. Who is culpable for a mistake made through the use of an AI program? We are in the nascent stages of this field, and there are unique cases with no legal precedents [15]. Moreover, no matter how much more accurate AI tools can be compared to their human counterparts, there is the possibility of misinterpreting data through false positives and negatives. Other major issues in legal culpability—for example, the processing of sensitive personal information and data collection, consent regarding processing, de-identification and pseudonymization, transparency, storage, and deletion—highlight the complex web that can obscure who or what is responsible. The human element is an important factor in incorporating AI in hospitals and pathology. Even if the process is completely automated with a routine digital imaging system and database management, human agreement will likely be essential at key points during any AI-patient-clinician encounter. Yet another hurdle is the investment of time and manpower to validate model datasets; as deep learning AI identifies patterns, the data used to train the AI model must be annotated and validated by medical specialists, creating additional costs and requiring considerable time to perfect an AI model that can be deployed with confidence to assist in medical practice. AI in legal domain will more likely have an immediate impact in the automation of the search of legal cases and literature, saving the time-consuming and tedious effort of junior lawyers and legal assistants burning the midnight oil.

At present, the most promising AI solutions in cancer or healthcare are laboriously built and limited in solving one well-defined and narrow problem at a time. Competition revolves around research into increasingly sophisticated and general AI toolkits. AI is presenting the cancer community with an opportunity to rethink the future disease management and continual of care models to cancer patients both inside and outside the hospital walls. The aspiration is to create AI systems that partner with oncologists and physicians across multiple disciplines and turn what today's just a powerful software toolkit into an infrastructure enabling value-based cancer care and cost-effective care delivery.

However, like many other new technologies coming into healthcare, AI faces trials that include regulatory barriers, interoperability issues with legacy databases, the availability of quality training data, considerable annotation efforts to generate reliable training data, security and patient privacy, and limitations regarding access to the crucial medical data as well as nonmedical data required to build powerful cancer-focused algorithms in the first place. Regardless, these obstacles are not impeding innovation, and healthcare stakeholders are realizing that unlocking AI's full potential necessitates strategic partnerships, quality data, and a sober understanding of statistics and return on investment. This involves the establishment of a quality and secured data infrastructure, clear policy, a thorough understanding of legal barriers and ramifications, and a strong commitment between care providers and technology vendors to mine data jointly, using AI to improve outcomes, reduce costs, and generate value. An AI revolution may be happening for those specialties already embracing digital operations such as radiology and healthcare information technology; however, it will take some time for others, such as pathology, to catch up due to the lack of digitized infrastructure and the previously discussed issues related to clinical procedures. Should these conundrums be addressed, AI could prove to be an incredibility powerful tool for improving the practice and productivity of oncologists and imaging specialists.

References

1. Searle J. Minds, brains, and programs. Behav Brain Sci. 1980;3:417–24.
2. Searle J. Minds, brains, and science. Cambridge, MA: Harvard University Press; 1984.
3. McCulloch WS, Pitts WH. A logical calculus of the ideas immanent in nervous activity. Bull Math Biophys. 1943;5:115–33.
4. Turing AM. "Computing Machinery and Intelligence" from Mind LIX, no. 2236, 1950:433–460.

5. Kleene SC. Representation of events in nerve nets and finite automata. In: Shannon C, McCarthy J, editors. Automata studies. Princeton: Princeton University Press; 1956. p. 3–41.
6. Moor J. The Dartmouth College artificial intelligence conference: the next fifty years. AI Mag. 2006;27:87–9.
7. Solomonoff RJ. The time scale of artificial intelligence: reflections on social effects. Hum Syst Manag. 1985;5:149–53.
8. Kurzweil R. The singularity is near. New York: Viking Press; 2005.
9. Winston PH, Prendergast KA. The AI business: the commercial uses of artificial intelligence. Cambridge, MA: MIT Press; 1985.
10. Barr A, Feigenbaum EA. The handbook of artificial intelligence, vol. 2. Los Altos: William Kaufmann; 1982.
11. Cohen PR, Feigenbaum EA. The handbook of artificial intelligence, vol. 3. Los Altos: William Kaufmann; 1982.
12. Mukherjee S. A.I. versus M.D. The New Yorker. https://www.newyorker.com/magazine/2017/04/03/ai-versus-md. Accessed 12 Mar 2018.
13. Goodfellow I, Bengio Y, Courville A. Deep learning (adaptive computation and machine learning series). Cambridge, MA: MIT Press; 2016.
14. Brynjolfsson E, Mcafee A. The second machine age: work, progress and prosperity in a time of brilliant technologies. New York: W.W. Norton & Company Inc; 2014.
15. Wong ST. Is pathology prepared for the adoption of artificial intelligence? Cancer Cytopathol. 2018;126:373–5.
16. Norris J, Joyce T, Tolman G. Silicon Valley Bank trends in healthcare investments and exits report. Santa Clara, CA; 2018.
17. Ahmed AM, et al. Augmented intelligence the next frontier [white paper] https://global.agfa-healthcare.com/int/ai/.
18. Pantanowitz L, Valenstein PN, et al. Review of the current state of whole slide imaging in pathology. J Pathol Inform. 2011;2:36.
19. US Food and Drug Administration. FDA allows marketing of first whole slide imaging system for digital pathology [FDA news release]. https://www.fda.gov/newsevents/newsroom/pressannouncements/ducm552742.htm.
20. Holzinger A, Malle B, et al. Towards the augmented pathologist: challenges of explainable-AI in digital pathology. arXiv: 1712.06657v1. 2017.

Chapter 9
The Hippies Were Right: Diet and Cancer Risk

Renee E. Stubbins and Eric H. Bernicker

Introduction

Dietary recommendations seem to change as often as the weather. Yet among the explosion of the general populations' belt line and the frequent grumbling that "experts" can't make up their mind regarding the best diet, there is an emerging consensus on what constitutes a healthy diet. And this healthy diet does not only decrease the risk of diabetes and heart disease but the most feared killer: cancer. And furthermore, this diet would also be better for the planet and future biodiversity of the planet.

The most recent report from the American Association for Cancer Research listed its top preventable causes of cancer, and among the top six causes are obesity/overweight, physical inactivity, and poor dietary choices, all of which are part of adapting a healthier lifestyle [1]. Lifestyle is very impactful on overall health, specifically people who eat poorly and do not exercise are likely to gain weight and become obese. Not only does obesity increase your risk of developing cancer but several other comorbidities as well (diabetes, heart disease, hypertension, etc.). Overall, the incidence of cancer is rising, and its increase is multifactorial [2]: (1) We are getting better at detecting and screening for certain cancers (breast, cervical,

R. E. Stubbins (✉)
Houston Methodist Cancer Center, Houston, TX, USA
e-mail: restubbins@houstonmethodist.org

E. H. Bernicker
Thoracic Medical Oncology, Cancer Center, Houston Methodist Hospital, Houston, TX, USA

Associate Professor of Clinical Medicine, Weill Cornell Medical College, New York, NY, USA

Associate Clinical Member, Houston Methodist Research Institute, Houston, TX, USA

Houston Methodist Cancer Center, Houston, TX, USA

© Springer Nature Switzerland AG 2019
E. H. Bernicker (ed.), *Cancer and Society*,
https://doi.org/10.1007/978-3-030-05855-5_9

prostate, colon, etc.). (2) People are living longer. (3) Our diets and lifestyle have become harmful; this chapter will focus on the latter.

The Link Between Dietary Intake and Cancer

The link between diet and cancer is complicated and is influenced by many factors. Human diets are complex and have many components: (1) *Macronutrients* are the major source of calories and primarily consist of carbohydrates, protein, and fat. (2) *Micronutrients* include vitamins and minerals in small amounts (hence the name micro). (3) *Phytonutrients* are nutrients found predominately in plants and are thought to serve as "protectors" against human disease and illness. The above nutrients can be obtained by consuming both animal- and plant-based foods; however, the cost and benefits we receive in our food choices can impact our health, including our risk of developing cancer.

The Cost of Consuming Animals

Animal-based foods can be further categorized into dairy and meat. Dairy products are a good source of protein, vitamin D, and calcium; they can be full-fat, low-fat, or nonfat. There remains quite a bit of controversy on whether there is a link between dairy and cancer, specifically high-fat dairy products have been linked to breast cancer [3] and ovarian cancer [4], but a recent review suggested that dairy products may reduce the risk to colon cancer [5]. Dairy consumption generally decreases as people age, partly due to the inability to make lactase, but conversely meat consumption typically increases.

Meat consists of mostly protein and fat along with iron, zinc, vitamins B1, B6, niacin, and B12. Both the American Cancer Society and American Institute for Cancer Research agree that red meat should be consumed in moderation; red meat consists of beef, lamb, veal, venison, bison, and pork. Additionally, both organizations recommend to avoid processed meats, which include lunch meat, bacon, sausage, salami, etc. [6, 7]. The International Agency for Research on Cancer (IARC) has classified processed meat as carcinogenic to humans and red meat as probably carcinogenic [8]. Several studies have shown that red meat consumption could be a leading cause of different types of cancer (pancreatic cancer, prostate cancer, and bladder cancer) [9–13], but their findings are not conclusive since there are conflicting studies [14, 15]. However, the relationship between red and processed meat consumption and CRC risk is well reviewed [16–19]. Analysis of 10 prospective studies showed a significant relationship between red and processed meat consumptions and risk to colorectal cancer (CRC); specifically it was estimated that daily consumption of 100 g of red meat daily increased the risk by 17% and daily consumption of 50 g or processed meats increased CRC risk by 18% [20]. There are numerous proposed mechanisms for explaining the relationship between red meat consumption and CRC, but we will focus on the following predominant mechanisms: heme iron in red meat, heterocyclic amines (HCAs), polycyclic aromatic hydrocarbons (PAHs) formed when cooking meat, and N-nitroso compounds (NOCs).

Red meat derives its color from heme iron found in the myoglobin in the muscles of the animal. It has been documented in both epidemiological [21, 22] and experimental studies [23] that heme iron can act as a carcinogen through various pathways: formation of N-nitroso compounds, lipid peroxidation, and cytotoxicity [24–26]. HCAs and PAHs are formed when cooking meats at very high temperatures, barbecuing or smoking [27, 28]. HCAs are formed when the nutrients from red meat react at high temperatures. PAHs are formed when the juices from the fat from the grilled meat drip onto the surface or fire, causing flames and smoke; this smoke can contain PAHs that may adhere to the surface of the meat. Thus, PAHs are also formed during other food preparation processes, such as smoking of meats [27]. There are very few epidemiological studies reviewing the relationship between HCAs and PAHs, partly because of the multiple variables involved (i.e., type of meat used, length of cooking, and temperature). There are a few animal studies that have established a link between high intake of HCAs and PAHs and cancer risk, but their relevance to the general population is questionable due to the excessive high amounts used in the studies [29]. Thus, additional studies are needed to fully understand the carcinogenicity of red/processed meats caused by HCAs and PAHs. Lastly, NOCs are obtained either through exogenous or endogenous routes: Exogenous NOCs typically source from tobacco products, diet (processed meats), and drugs [30, 31]. Endogenous NOCs are formed when nitrates react with products of degraded amino acids [32]. Certain NOCs are capable of interacting with alkylating agents and causing DNA damage potentially increasing the risk to CRC [33]. In summary, HCAs, PAHs, and NOCs are mutagens and animal carcinogens that have serious costs to our health if consumed in excess. To help overcome the potential "costs" of consuming meat and its possible carcinogens, experts have strongly suggested including more plant-based foods in the diet.

The Benefit of Consuming Plants

Plant-based foods consist of macro/micronutrients and phytonutrients. Epidemiological and experimental studies have consistently shown that a diet high in plant foods is correlated with a lower risk to various cancers [34]. Specifically, "the evidence for a protective effect of greater vegetable and fruit consumption is consistent for cancers of the stomach, esophagus, lung, oral cavity and pharynx, endometrium, pancreas, and colon" [34]. They further elaborated on the specific nutrients that could play a protective role against cancer (dithiolthiones, isothiocyanates, indole-32-carbinol, allium compounds, isoflavones, protease inhibitors, saponins, phytosterols, inositol hexaphosphate, vitamin C, D-limonene, lutein, folic acid, beta-carotene (and other carotenoids), lycopene, selenium, vitamin E, flavonoids, and dietary fiber). Moreover, other experimental studies have confirmed that this protective effect against cancer is not due to one single nutrient but largely related to the high amount of phytonutrients found in plant-based foods; therefore variety is important [35]. There are over 25,000 phytonutrients found in plants, and many can protect us from carcinogenesis by preventing or inhibiting cancer initiation and progression [36]. These phytonutrients (vitamins C and E and carotenoids) can act as antioxidants by scavenging for reactive oxygen species preventing DNA damage or lipid peroxidation [37]. Additionally, phytonutrients have been shown to affect pro-inflammatory cell signaling and gene expression [38]. Lastly, there is an overwhelming amount of evidence and research on the benefits of fiber (insoluble and soluble) in your diet and reducing cancer risk. The mechanisms by which fiber protects our cells from damage are numerous and beyond the scope of this chapter. However, a popular and well-documented theory is that high amounts of fiber in our diet cause us to defecate often and consistently, therefore decreasing the time carcinogens are exposed to our colon [39]. As plant-based foods are considered one of the richest and a sole source of our dietary fiber, including them in the diet is going to have a protective effect.

There is a strong consensus among the scientific community that eating more plant-based foods is associated with lower risk to multiple human diseases (obesity, diabetes, heart disease, and cancer). It is hard to find a negative or "cost" to eating too many fruits and vegetables. You can achieve a well-balanced diet by becoming a vegetarian or vegan versus omnivores who are forced to balance their meat intake to make sure their health cost-benefit ratio is in their favor.

The Link Between Factory Farming and Pollution

Many people do not give much thought to how their food is raised and slaughtered. As the old saying goes, if slaughter houses were made of glass, most people would be vegetarians. Most of our animal products (eggs, milk, and meat) come from factory farms. There are several documentaries that have recently researched and carefully documented how "factory farming" is both inhumane for the animals (and for slaughterhouse workers) and the environmental consequences that arise as a result of massive concentration of animals and their waste. The formal definition for factory farming is "a system of rearing livestock using intensive methods, by which poultry, pigs, or cattle are confined indoors under strictly controlled conditions." When animals are confined in this tight space and are fed in excess to make them grow faster (in order to shorten the time to get their body parts to the market), the waste output (i.e., manure) is going to be impressive. This excess waste is not only harmful to the animals and workers; it has been shown to cause water and air contamination [40–43]. Furthermore, the living conditions for these animals are breeding grounds for "super bugs" or methicillin-resistant *Staphylococcus aureus* (MRSA) bacterium.

MRSA is becoming an overwhelming problem for healthcare facilities; a study in the Netherlands found that more than 20% of their MRSA cases were caused by "livestock origin" MRSA [44]. The generation of this MRSA bacterium are multifactorial, but the most influential factor is the use of antibiotics to treat the animals. Factory farm animals again are in confined spaces and are more likely to become sick because of their living conditions (too much manure) so antibiotics are used because it is the most cost-effective way to maintain or improve the animal's health and feed efficiency [45, 46].

Factory farming not only takes a toll on health but the environment as well. The excessive waste products from factory farms can affect our soil, air, and water resources. Animal waste is not treated like human waste and is often used in excess to "fertilize" the soil of the farmlands; this overfertilization smothers the soil and reduces its fertility. Additionally, animal waste carries with it high amounts of methane and hydrogen sulfide, where both contribute to global warming and can potentially harm the workers and others living nearby. Lastly, the chemical fertilizers, excess animal waste, and pesticides can contaminate the water runoff from the factory farm affecting local water resources, animals, and plants.

Before the industrialization of farming, farmers and the land had a balanced relationship. The farmers would use the "farmer's almanac" and rotate their crops and graze their animals. The grazing animals would naturally fertilize the land, and the soil's fertility and vitality would be maintained. Although health-conscious individuals are choosing to eat less animal products, the world as a whole is eating more meat; thus we are changing our climate as a result of our dietary choices [47].

The Link Between Dietary Choices and Climate Change

Global warming is becoming a pressing concern, and greenhouse gases (GHG) are a major cause; specifically our current agriculture practices are significantly adding to the increase in atmospheric methane and nitrous oxide. Our food choices not only affect our health but our environment as well. Studies have shown that meals similar in nutritional value may vary by a factor of 2–9 in their GHGs [48, 49].

Specifically, this variation depends on the amount of processing of the animal or plant, amount of nitrogen fertilizer used, soil and manure usage, fermentation from the animals, transportation, and the storage of the food items.

As meat becomes more industrialized and less expensive to produce, the cost of meat becomes more affordable to lower-income families and to developing countries. Our current trends in food choices are leading to more costly environmental effects [50]. However, preliminary studies suggest that switching to a Mediterranean or diets that are mostly plant-based with small amount animal-based foods are more sustainable for the environment [51].

Thus, while eating meat clearly affects an individual's health risk (and thus many people argue that it is a personal decision), the terrible environmental cost can be considered as a significant risk factor in much the same way as secondhand smoke is. In fact, advocates can learn much from the way in which the realization that secondhand cigarette smoke posed risks to non-smokers (innocent bystanders) made a tremendous difference in the societal discussion of cigarette smoking in public. Likewise, the decision to eat meat in many ways produces the "secondhand smoke" of methane emissions from cattle. Raising animals for slaughter and consumption is a significant anthropogenic contributor to methane emissions [52, 53]. Agribusiness is one of the world's worst polluters, as manure from incarcerated animals, pesticides, and antibiotics often run off and pollute streams. And of course, shipping animals to slaughter houses and then meat packages to markets also raises the carbon footprint.

And it is not just the waste from these large concentrations of animals and the massive GHG's they release that adds to the risk of further climate change. Huge amounts of forest have to be cut down in order to have land to graze or land to grow crops—that will be later fed to animals. Worldwide, deforestation is a major contributor to both climate change as well as a major cause of loss of biodiversity [54]. While watching nature specials might lead children to assume that there are still many places in the world where exotic animals run free and frolic in the sun, the vast majority of animals in the world are raised for slaughter and human consumption [55].

While dietary changes clearly are not fully protective against developing cancers, we think that major research bodies have not emphasized enough the harmful effects of meat consumption (and not just red meat: poultry and pork production and consumption carry as much potential harm to patients and the environment as beef). As more data is generated on the role of the microbiome in health and disease, it is becoming clear that the bacterial populations inhabiting the human gut differ between vegetarians and meat eaters and the latter have more bacterial populations associated with an inflammatory signature [56, 57]. This is not only important for the development of colorectal cancer but in fact might also influence how patients subsequently respond to immunotherapy drugs such as immune checkpoint inhibitors should they develop cancer [58].

Proposed Solutions

As we have reviewed the literature thus far in this chapter, it is obvious that our current diet trends are costing us more than our personal health but also the health of our climate. An obvious solution is for us to adapt a more plant-based diet; however, as healthcare providers we know that simply recommending a diet to a patient is not enough to get them to change their lifestyle. Thus, we should focus on educating our patients and proposing realistic and feasible solutions. For example, explaining "the why" about our recommendations and offering them a detailed explanation of the benefits of a primarily plant-based diet. Additionally, if the patient insists on having animal-based foods in their diet, explaining the benefits of sustainable farming and the benefits of shopping at a local farmer's market vs. major grocery stores. Lastly, it is important that we continue to educate ourselves and other healthcare professionals. As chronic diseases continue to rise, hindering their severity by educating individuals in healthcare is our first line of defense in preventing epidemics.

We need to continue to press major medical groups to take a more forceful stand on plant-based nutrition, both as a way to benefit human health and to protect the environment. We need to support efforts to introduce more plant-based diets in schools so that children are exposed to healthier diets in their formative years. Healthcare workers need to help push to end beef subsidies and other legislation that makes it a crime to expose what actually happens in slaughterhouses (so called Ag-gag laws). Cancer survivors also need to be encouraged to adopt meat-free diets even if their cancer was not one that is classically associated with meat eating; recent data showed that breast cancer survivors who kept eating meat had worse outcomes [59].

The shelves of many grocery stores are filled with dietary supplements that patients frequently turn to in order to prevent or treat illness. But the reality is that the data on the benefits of supplements to prevent cancer is poor at best [60]. Patients should be encouraged to save their money on unproven supplements and instead eat a diet with greater amounts of fruits and vegetables.

Lastly, healthcare workers need to help patients focus on how the food on their plates affects the health of their communities and planet. Climate change and environmental pollution are not only driven by fossil fuel companies and industrial production: the way we produce animals has a great deal of impact on the quality of our environment and the future climate our descendants will inherit. By educating and encouraging our patients to adopt a plant-based diet, we will give them ways to increase their own health as well as the health of the biosphere.

References

1. Research A.A.f.C. AACR cancer progress report. American Association of Cancer Research: Philadelphia, PA. 2017.
2. Institute N.C. Cancer statistics. National Institutes of Health; National Cancer Institute. Bethesda, MD. 2017.
3. Kroenke CH, et al. High- and low-fat dairy intake, recurrence, and mortality after breast cancer diagnosis. J Natl Cancer Inst. 2013;105(9):616–23.
4. Larsson SC, Orsini N, Wolk A. Milk, milk products and lactose intake and ovarian cancer risk: a meta-analysis of epidemiological studies. Int J Cancer. 2006;118(2):431–41.
5. Aune D, et al. Dairy products and colorectal cancer risk: a systematic review and meta-analysis of cohort studies. Ann Oncol. 2012;23(1):37–45.
6. Society AC. Cancer prevention & early detection: facts & figures 2017–2018. Atlanta: American Cancer Society; 2017.
7. Wiseman M. The second World Cancer Research Fund/American Institute for Cancer Research expert report. Food, nutrition, physical activity, and the prevention of cancer: a global perspective. Proc Nutr Soc. 2008;67(3):253–6.
8. Bouvard V, et al. Carcinogenicity of consumption of red and processed meat. Lancet Oncol. 2015;16(16):1599–600.
9. Butler C, et al. Diet and the risk of head-and-neck cancer among never-smokers and smokers in a Chinese population. Cancer Epidemiol. 2017;46:20–6.
10. Caini S, et al. Food of animal origin and risk of non-Hodgkin lymphoma and multiple myeloma: a review of the literature and meta-analysis. Crit Rev Oncol Hematol. 2016;100:16–24.

11. Lippi G, Mattiuzzi C, Cervellin G. Meat consumption and cancer risk: a critical review of published meta-analyses. Crit Rev Oncol Hematol. 2016;97:1–14.
12. Wu K, et al. Associations between unprocessed red and processed meat, poultry, seafood and egg intake and the risk of prostate cancer: a pooled analysis of 15 prospective cohort studies. Int J Cancer. 2016;138(10):2368–82.
13. Wolk A. Potential health hazards of eating red meat. J Intern Med. 2017;281(2):106–22.
14. Li F, et al. Red and processed meat intake and risk of bladder cancer: a meta-analysis. Int J Clin Exp Med. 2014;7(8):2100–10.
15. Bylsma LC, Alexander DD. A review and meta-analysis of prospective studies of red and processed meat, meat cooking methods, heme iron, heterocyclic amines and prostate cancer. Nutr J. 2015;14:125.
16. Willett WC, et al. Relation of meat, fat, and fiber intake to the risk of colon cancer in a prospective study among women. N Engl J Med. 1990;323(24):1664–72.
17. Bostick RM, et al. Sugar, meat, and fat intake, and non-dietary risk factors for colon cancer incidence in Iowa women (United States). Cancer Causes Control. 1994;5(1):38–52.
18. Goldbohm RA, et al. A prospective cohort study on the relation between meat consumption and the risk of colon cancer. Cancer Res. 1994;54(3):718–23.
19. Giovannucci E, et al. Relationship of diet to risk of colorectal adenoma in men. J Natl Cancer Inst. 1992;84(2):91–8.
20. Chan DS, et al. Red and processed meat and colorectal cancer incidence: meta-analysis of prospective studies. PLoS One. 2011;6(6):e20456.
21. Bastide NM, Pierre FH, Corpet DE. Heme iron from meat and risk of colorectal cancer: a meta-analysis and a review of the mechanisms involved. Cancer Prev Res (Phila). 2011;4(2):177–84.
22. Fonseca-Nunes A, Jakszyn P, Agudo A. Iron and cancer risk–a systematic review and meta-analysis of the epidemiological evidence. Cancer Epidemiol Biomark Prev. 2014;23(1):12–31.
23. Sesink AL, et al. Red meat and colon cancer: the cytotoxic and hyperproliferative effects of dietary heme. Cancer Res. 1999;59(22):5704–9.
24. Tappel A. Heme of consumed red meat can act as a catalyst of oxidative damage and could initiate colon, breast and prostate cancers, heart disease and other diseases. Med Hypotheses. 2007;68(3):562–4.
25. Bingham SA, Hughes R, Cross AJ. Effect of white versus red meat on endogenous N-nitrosation in the human colon and further evidence of a dose response. J Nutr. 2002;132(11 Suppl):3522S–5S.
26. Toyokuni S. Role of iron in carcinogenesis: cancer as a ferrotoxic disease. Cancer Sci. 2009;100(1):9–16.
27. Cross AJ, Sinha R. Meat-related mutagens/carcinogens in the etiology of colorectal cancer. Environ Mol Mutagen. 2004;44(1):44–55.
28. Jägerstad M, Skog K. Genotoxicity of heat-processed foods. Mutat Res. 2005;574(1–2):156–72.
29. Sugimura T, et al. Heterocyclic amines: mutagens/carcinogens produced during cooking of meat and fish. Cancer Sci. 2004;95(4):290–9.
30. Scanlan RA. Formation and occurrence of nitrosamines in food. Cancer Res. 1983;43(5 Suppl):2435s–40s.
31. Mirvish SS. Role of N-nitroso compounds (NOC) and N-nitrosation in etiology of gastric, esophageal, nasopharyngeal and bladder cancer and contribution to cancer of known exposures to NOC. Cancer Lett. 1995;93(1):17–48.
32. Tricker AR. N-nitroso compounds and man: sources of exposure, endogenous formation and occurrence in body fluids. Eur J Cancer Prev. 1997;6(3):226–68.
33. Bos JL. Ras oncogenes in human cancer: a review. Cancer Res. 1989;49(17):4682–9.
34. Steinmetz KA, Potter JD. Vegetables, fruit, and cancer prevention: a review. J Am Diet Assoc. 1996;96(10):1027–39.
35. Chen H, Liu RH. Potential mechanisms of action of dietary phytochemicals for cancer prevention by targeting cellular signaling transduction pathways. J Agric Food Chem. 2018;66(13):3260–76.

36. Béliveau R, Gingras D. Role of nutrition in preventing cancer. Can Fam Physician. 2007;53(11):1905–11.
37. Byers T, Perry G. Dietary carotenes, vitamin C, and vitamin E as protective antioxidants in human cancers. Annu Rev Nutr. 1992;12:139–59.
38. Surh YJ. NF-kappa B and Nrf2 as potential chemopreventive targets of some anti-inflammatory and antioxidative phytonutrients with anti-inflammatory and antioxidative activities. Asia Pac J Clin Nutr. 2008;17(Suppl 1):269–72.
39. Fuchs CS, et al. Dietary fiber and the risk of colorectal cancer and adenoma in women. N Engl J Med. 1999;340(3):169–76.
40. Ferguson DD, et al. Detection of airborne methicillin-resistant Staphylococcus aureus inside and downwind of a swine building, and in animal feed: potential occupational, animal health, and environmental implications. J Agromedicine. 2016;21(2):149–53.
41. Springer B, et al. Methicillin-resistant Staphylococcus aureus: a new zoonotic agent? Wien Klin Wochenschr. 2009;121(3–4):86–90.
42. van Cleef BA, et al. Livestock-associated MRSA in household members of pig farmers: transmission and dynamics of carriage, a prospective cohort study. PLoS One. 2015;10(5):e0127190.
43. Parris K. Impact of agriculture on water pollution in OECD countries: recent trends and future prospects. Int J Water Resour Dev. 2011;27(1):33–52.
44. van Loo I, et al. Emergence of methicillin-resistant Staphylococcus aureus of animal origin in humans. Emerg Infect Dis. 2007;13(12):1834–9.
45. Dibner JJ, Richards JD. Antibiotic growth promoters in agriculture: history and mode of action. Poult Sci. 2005;84(4):634–43.
46. Cromwell GL. Why and how antibiotics are used in swine production. Anim Biotechnol. 2002;13(1):7–27.
47. Delgado CL. Rising consumption of meat and milk in developing countries has created a new food revolution. J Nutr. 2003;133(11 Suppl 2):3907S–10S.
48. Carlsson-Kanyama A. Climate change and dietary choices — how can emissions of greenhouse gases from food consumption be reduced? Food Policy. 1998;23(3–4):277–93.
49. Engström, et al. Environmental assessment of Swedish agriculture. Ecol Econ. 2007;60(3):550–63.
50. Carlsson-Kanyama A, Linden A-L. Trends in food production and consumption: Swedish experiences from environmental and cultural impacts. Int J Sustain Dev. 2001;4(4):392.
51. Duchin F. A world trade model based on comparative advantage with m regions, n goods, and k factors. Econ Syst Res. 2005;17(2):141–62.
52. Steinfeld H, Gerber P. Livestock production and the global environment: consume less or produce better? Proc Natl Acad Sci U S A. 2010;107(43):18237–8.
53. Wang Y, et al. Mitigating greenhouse gas and Ammonia emissions from swine manure management: a system analysis. Environ Sci Technol. 2017;51(8):4503–11.
54. Alroy J. Effects of habitat disturbance on tropical forest biodiversity. Proc Natl Acad Sci U S A. 2017;114(23):6056–61.
55. Harari YN. Industrial Farming is one of the worst crimes in history. The Guardian. 2015.
56. do Rosario VA, Fernandes R, Trindade EB. Vegetarian diets and gut microbiota: important shifts in markers of metabolism and cardiovascular disease. Nutr Rev. 2016;74(7):444–54.
57. Franco-de-Moraes AC, et al. Worse inflammatory profile in omnivores than in vegetarians associates with the gut microbiota composition. Diabetol Metab Syndr. 2017;9:62.
58. Bhatt AP, Redinbo MR, Bultman SJ. The role of the microbiome in cancer development and therapy. CA Cancer J Clin. 2017;67(4):326–44.
59. Parada H, et al. Grilled, barbecued, and smoked meat intake and survival following breast cancer. J Natl Cancer Inst. 2017;109(6):djw299.
60. Manson JE, Bassuk SS. Vitamin and mineral supplements: what clinicians need to know. JAMA. 2018;319(9):859–60.

Chapter 10
Protons and Prejudice: Finding Sense and Sensibility in the Development of a Costly Medical Therapy

Andrew M. Farach

History of Proton Therapy in the United States

Throughout history, war, for all its atrocities, has contributed vastly to the advancement of medicine. Stemming from work on the Manhattan Project during WWII, physicists developed high-energy particle accelerators such as the cyclotron that could be utilized in the treatment of human disease. The first proposed use of high-energy protons for cancer therapy was described in 1946 by Dr. Robert R. Wilson in a seminal paper entitled "Radiological Use of Fast Protons." In this paper, Dr. Wilson describes the properties of high-energy photons as making it possible to "irradiate intensely a strictly localized region within the body, with but little skin dose. Precision exposure of well-defined small volumes in the body will soon be feasible" [1].

Soon, as it turned out, would not come until 1954 when the first patient was treated at the Berkeley Radiation Laboratory in California. While experimental treatments continued for thousands of patients, proton beam therapy (PBT) would not become an FDA-approved medical device until 1988. Loma Linda University became the first hospital-based proton center in 1990 prompting a rapid adoption of this expensive technology at many centers across the United States. Despite no randomized data to support a clinical benefit or cost-effectiveness, a proton center arms race began with promises of improved clinical outcomes over conventional radiation therapy.

A. M. Farach (✉)
Radiation Oncology, Houston Methodist Hospital, Houston, TX, USA
e-mail: amfarach@houstonmethodist.org

© Springer Nature Switzerland AG 2019
E. H. Bernicker (ed.), *Cancer and Society*,
https://doi.org/10.1007/978-3-030-05855-5_10

The Allure of Protons: Something to Brag About

To understand this rapid proliferation of proton facilities, one must first understand the basics of the technology. Radiation of all types works by creating DNA damage in both cancer cells and normal tissues. Delivering radiation therapy over a series of weeks, *fractionation*, helps to accumulate damage to cancer cells more than normal healthy cells. Over 60% of all cancer patients will receive radiation therapy at some point in their treatment course. Protons are heavy subatomic particles that carry a positive charge, while photons are high-energy X-rays with no mass and no charge. For this reason, they interact differently with tissues in the body.

PBT is an attractive alternative to traditional photon therapy because of the physical differences in how dose is absorbed in the body. The allure of PBT is based on two widely accepted presumptions: radiation damages normal tissue, and radiation damage is directly related to the volume and dose received by that normal tissue [2]. A critical component of radiation oncology training is learning the dose and volume tolerances of normal tissues to radiation. A comprehensive knowledge of dose tolerance and fractionation allows the radiation oncologist to maximize dosage to a given tumor while keeping the risk of damage to normal tissues low. This is typically referred to as the therapeutic ratio. Maximizing this ratio is always the goal, to destroy cancer tissue and cause minimal damage to nearby normal tissue.

The field of radiation oncology has embraced technology for decades in order to maximize the therapeutic ratio and allow for dose escalation in order to improve the chance of cure. A great example is the development of a technique called stereotactic body radiation therapy (SBRT). SBRT was developed by harnessing technological advancements in diagnostic imaging, immobilization, image guidance, dose calculation algorithms, and linear accelerator design. With this technique, large ablative doses of photons (and potentially protons) are delivered precisely to tumors in just 3–5 days. With this precision, only a few millimeters of normal tissue margin receive high doses of radiation. Since its adoption in the early 2000s, SBRT has dramatically improved survival rates for inoperable or elderly patients with early-stage lung cancer [3].

Technologies such as intensity-modulated radiation therapy (IMRT) and image-guided radiation therapy (IGRT) also have improved outcomes with photons in many tumor sites, resulting in lower rates of short-term and long-term side effects. The concept of IMRT is similar to that of shining multiple magnifying glasses on an ant. Multiple beams of high-energy photons converge on a single target and minimize the effect of any one beam on healthy tissues. Given that side effects are most likely to occur in high-dose regions, IMRT uses computer algorithms to optimize or modulate the dose of radiation. This allows the physician to set limits of radiation dose on sensitive organs and reduce the probability of side effects. The benefit, however, comes at the cost of dramatically increased low- and intermediate-dose radiation spread in the normal tissues around the tumor, *integral dose*. As photons are X-rays and pass easily through the body, dose is delivered almost evenly along the beam path. This is referred to as *entrance dose* (in front of the target) and *exit dose* (behind the target). By utilizing multiple beam angles, high-dose regions can be controlled; however more normal tissue is exposed to low or intermediate radiation dose. The long-term impact of this intermediate radiation exposure has yet to be fully demonstrated.

As IMRT cost is significantly higher than 3D conformal radiation therapy (a technique that typically utilized fewer beam angles and does not incorporate computer optimization), numerous comparative effectiveness (phase III) trials were performed to demonstrate the clinical benefit of IMRT and to justify the expense. Owing to vast improvements in high-dose region control over 3D techniques, IMRT represented a leap forward for the field of radiation oncology. This benefit is clearly supported in the literature for certain cancer types such as head and neck cancer. In short, the theory that improved control over high-dose radiation would result in less side effects was easily proven to be true for IMRT.

With PBT, entrance dose is significantly less than that of photons. Protons are charged particles and at high energies do not interact significantly with tissue. This results in minimal absorbed entrance dose. As protons pass through tissue they slow; the energy lost is inversely proportional to the square of their velocity ultimately resulting in a massive release of energy in a narrow range and at a specific depth in the body. This is termed the *Bragg peak*. With PBT there is essentially no exit dose beyond this peak representing a unique and favorable dose profile that can be exploited to reduce doses to normal tissue along the beam path. With PBT the integral dose seen with IMRT is significantly reduced. This improved dose control theoretically allows for dose escalation and improved chances of cure with equal or lesser side effects.

Given the interaction profile of protons in tissue, they are ideally suited for tumors near critical anatomic structures with limited motion such as in the brain or spine and for growing children where even low doses of radiation can have pronounced long-term health impacts. Another potential benefit of PBT is in patients with genetic syndromes that predispose them to increased risk of radiation-induced malignancy. To the radiation oncology community, PBT represents an exciting emerging option and would provide another tool to improve outcomes for our patients. It is only rational to expect that data would support PBT over photon therapy in certain disease sites where there is a clear dosing advantage, similarly to the documented benefit seen with IMRT. One key distinction, however, is that control over high-dose regions with photons is excellent and unlikely to be improved upon with PBT. The improvement with PBT would be in the intermediate- to low-dose regions with less intense biologic effect. Because of this, it may be harder to demonstrate a dramatic clinical benefit.

If You Build It, They Might Come

The finances of delivering PBT are extraordinary. Most proton centers cost in excess of $150 million dollars to construct. A typical photon therapy machine, on the other hand, costs approximately $3 million. To distribute this up-front cost, university-based

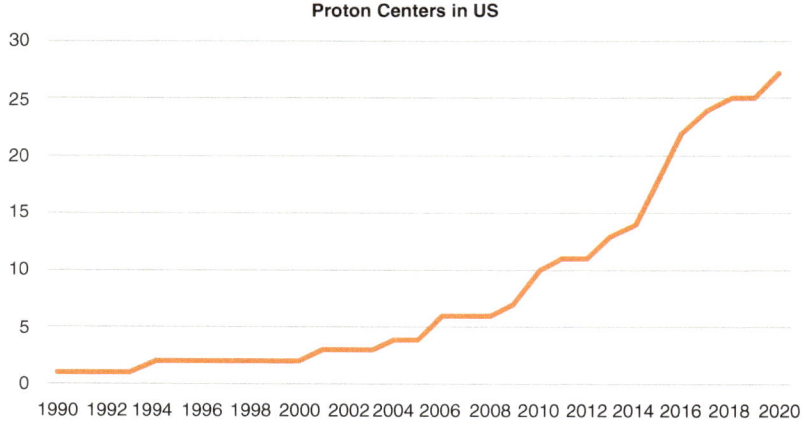

Fig. 10.1 Proton therapy centers are proliferating rapidly across the United States

proton centers have often partnered with for-profit private investors seeking an opportunity to cash in on the proton bubble. For instance, the University of Texas M.D. Anderson Proton Center, Houston, is a majority investor-owned, for-profit entity and does not fall under the umbrella of the University of Texas System. This financial structure was designed to protect the university's credit rating in the case of a financial shortfall. Since the mid-2000s, investors and top cancer centers have flocked to the PBT market resulting in a rapid proliferation of facilities across the United States (Fig. 10.1). Aiming to be first to market and with promises of annual revenue of more than $50 million, investors began pouring money into this potentially game-changing technology.

With smaller entrepreneurial ventures playing a large role in establishing proton facilities, the primary objective strayed away from conducting much-needed safety and efficacy research and shifted to return on investment. With operating expenses ranging from $15 to 25 million per year and reimbursement of around $40,000 per patient, high patient volumes and reliable insurance payments were required to avoid substantial losses. Proton centers began extending hours, often treating through the night and early in the morning to keep volume high. For some, that might mean receiving 8 weeks of daily PBT at 2 am! To minimize cost and maximize patient throughput, lower energy or fixed beam rooms were developed, posing a risk of suboptimal outcomes in certain cases given a lack of complexity in treatment planning capability.

Unfortunately for many of the investors in PBT, profit models were guided by the "Field of Dreams" principle: "if you build it, they will come." In many of the models, investors overestimated the number of patients that PBT would attract and failed to consider the importance of physician referrals. Dr. Peter Johnstone, former CEO of the failed Indiana University Proton Center, is quoted as saying "the biggest problem these guys have is extra capacity. They don't have enough patients to fill the rooms."

Speaking about his experience in Indiana, "we began to see that simply having a proton center didn't mean people would come" [4]. As a result of ambitious and overly optimistic patient volume estimates, numerous facilities have faced financial ruin including bankruptcy, defaults on debt, and multimillion dollar losses [4].

Lately, hospitals are turning to the municipal bond market to finance new PBT centers as private loans have become more difficult because of the previous financial failures. Municipal bonds often are tax-exempt and carry favorable interest rates so centers have moved quickly to this market for financing. In 2017 alone, municipal bonds issued $418 million of debt for proton centers across the United States [5]. This is compared to $239 million in the prior 10 years combined. This trend concerns some health policy researchers as the potential exists for a massive default once payments are due.

The greatest potential for improved outcomes with PBT exists for pediatric patients and for patients with rare brain, spine, skull base, or eye tumors. However, bottom-line financial pressures prompted the development of an artificial proton niche to market the technology to patients with more common diseases such as prostate cancer, despite no clear scientific or clinical merit to claims of superiority. To put it in perspective, nearly a quarter million American men are diagnosed with prostate cancer each year, while only four thousand children are diagnosed with brain tumors. Proton centers clearly would not survive on pediatric patients alone. Dr. Paul Levy put it best when he said, "The easiest group to market to in the country is a group of men worrying about the functioning of their penis" [6]. Despite controversy regarding overdiagnosis, overtreatment, and the benefits of prostate cancer screening, the protons-for-prostate marketing campaign forged ahead. "It is an example of how our health-care system is set up to become more expensive without getting necessarily better," said Steven Pearson, president of the Institute for Clinical and Economic Review, at the Massachusetts General Hospital [6].

Examining the Data Surrounding Protons for Prostate

Several trials were conducted to examine the benefit of radiation dose escalation in prostate cancer following a 2005 report of the combined experience from nine institutions [7]. This study demonstrated improvement in prostate cancer control at 5 years with higher doses of radiation, albeit with increased bladder and rectal dysfunction. Several single institution studies utilized IMRT in dose-escalated patients to reduce bowel and bladder doses. As a result, they demonstrated decreased side effects; however no randomized data was available. The RTOG 0126 study was published on October 8, 2013 after examining outcomes in patients treated with 3D conformal radiation therapy or IMRT [8]. In this study, patients treated with IMRT had significantly lower volumes of bladder and rectum receiving high doses of radiation, owing the improved control over high-dose areas with this technique. These reductions in normal tissue dose translated to a 26% reduction in significant bothersome rectal irritation. Severe side effects were rarely observed. A similar study was performed utilizing PBT as part of the treatment for dose escalation with a similar side-effect profile [9]. Of interest, there was no significant reduction in late-occurring bladder toxicity with IMRT as the bladder neck and prostatic urethra receive the full prescription dose in prostate radiation: by definition these cannot be spared. Based on this data, IMRT clearly warranted the increased cost of treatment.

In 2013, another important manuscript was published by Yale researchers comparing the use, cost, and early toxicity outcomes in Medicare patients receiving PBT or IMRT for prostate cancer in 2008/2009. In this study, among 27,647 men receiving radiation therapy for prostate cancer, 553 (2%) were treated with PBT. These patients tended to be white, younger, healthier, and more affluent than those receiving photons. The median reimbursement for PBT was $32,428 versus $18,575 for IMRT. Abstracting out from this data, if all men received PBT, the result would be an increased Medicare expenditure of $383 million to taxpayers solely for the treatment of prostate cancer. While there was a slight improvement in urinary symptoms at 6 months (9.5% vs 5.9%) favoring PBT, these differences disappeared by a year [10]. Similar results were seen in a prospective study conducted at the University of Pennsylvania and published in 2015 [10].

Based on results such as these, private insurance companies began denying coverage for PBT for prostate cancer. The Molina policy recommendation states that PBT is not medically necessary and may not be authorized due to lack of data to support improved outcomes over IMRT [11]. The American Society for Therapeutic Radiology and Oncology (ASTRO) states that the comparative efficacy research is ongoing and that PBT should only be offered in the context of a clinical trial or registry [12]. As a result, obtaining insurance coverage for PBT may be difficult for many patients or require a lengthy appeals process. These difficulties in coverage no doubt affect patient volumes at proton centers.

Proton Therapy in the United Kingdom

As a government-sponsored universal health-care system, the National Health Service (NHS) in the United Kingdom has taken a more cautious approach to the development of PBT. The NHS began paying for patients to receive PBT abroad in 2008 for select indications. The National Proton Beam Therapy Service Development Programme constructed a strategic outline for the development of a national PBT service with their initial publication in late 2012. In this publication, they examined the national demand for PBT and estimated that 1500 patients per year would benefit from PBT [13]. The population of the United Kingdom in 2012 was 63.7 million with nearly 150,000 requiring radiation therapy services. Essentially 1% of UK cancer patients were considered to benefit from PBT, none of which have prostate cancer. Using quality-adjusted life years, the lifetime benefit of PBT was estimated to be £1 billion. The NHS proposed a model to develop two proton centers to meet the clinical demand of the country with geographical access considered. This model would allow for full capacity treatment at each center and presumably result in a net financial gain, when compared to sending patients abroad for therapy. These proton centers are currently still in development with plans to open in Manchester in late 2018 and London in 2020.

Interestingly, there was no mention in this report about the potential for private proton facilities entering the market and no modeling of the financial impact on NHS facilities. In fact, in April 2018, a private facility operated by Proton Partners International became the first to treat a patient in the United Kingdom with high-energy PBT for…wait for it…prostate cancer. Proton Partners International plans to build eight centers in the United Kingdom and can treat patients at nearly half the current cost to the NHS of sending a patient abroad for treatment excluding travel and housing costs. Given that the NHS facilities have yet to open, this private group has negotiated contracts with the NHS to provide services to UK patients and will ultimately impact US-based treatment facilities previously profiting from out-sourced UK patients.

While the UK approach is clearly the more measured and financially sensible approach to implementing PBT, there are difficulties associated with such an approach, especially in our global capitalistic society. Medicine is far less paternal-istic than in the past, and patients often utilize the Internet to guide their care, for better or worse. As the NHS slowly and methodically develops proton centers in the United Kingdom, it is impossible to discount the perceived sacrifice citizens may feel on an individual scale. Parents of children with brain tumors diagnosed prior to the development of PBT in the United Kingdom had to transfer their care to another country where cultural differences, lack of family support, and lost wages may have a dramatic negative personal impact. These families, in certain situations, may be left with the difficult decision to travel for medicine or stay home and receive what may be an inferior therapy. Imagine the psychological strain that this decision might have on a parent of a child who experienced a poor outcome, lost hearing, decreased IQ, or impotence. There are also practical considerations. Brain tumors in children typically present because the patient is symptomatic and may require immediate neurosurgical intervention, for instance, to decrease pressure on the brain. Delays in gaining access to PBT may diminish the potential benefit of such a therapy. A parent living in an industrialized country, such as England, may reasonably wonder why the United Kingdom is 64 years behind the United States in treating a patient with PBT.

The Ashya King case poignantly highlighted this issue. In July 2014 at Southampton General Hospital in England, 5-year-old Ashya King was diagnosed with pediatric medulloblastoma, the most common primary brain tumor in children. This disease is probably the least controversial disease site for the theoretical benefit of PBT as radiation to the entire brain and spinal cord is a critical component for cure. However, based on the scientific literature available at that time, there was no demonstrable benefit to PBT over photon therapy. There was, however, clear evi-dence that treatment delay could result in shortened survival. Based on their knowl-edge of the data and specifics of Ashya's case, doctors at the hospital as well as the NHS Specialized Services Proton Clinical Reference Panel determined PBT would not benefit Ashya over conventional therapy. As a result, the family left the hospital against medical advice and boarded a ferry for France to get Ashya PBT. This action prompted an international manhunt for the family who was ultimately captured and arrested in Spain. An emergency court hearing allowed Ashya to be transferred to Prague where he would eventually receive PBT 8 weeks after his initial surgery.

There was a clear risk that such a transfer would significantly reduce the boy's chances of cure due to delays in the initiation of radiation therapy. Ashya's doctors in Southampton knew the results of the PNET 4 trial published in 2012 that clearly demonstrated that a treatment delay of 7 weeks resulted in a 5-year event-free survival of 67% compared to 81% for those treated promptly [14]. The general rule of thumb is to begin radiation treatment within 4 weeks of surgery. It was not until 2016 that a phase II trial reported potentially improved hearing preservation and equal survival for PBT over conventional photon therapy [15] in patients with pediatric medulloblastoma. However, the King family, armed with Internet access, felt strongly that PBT was the best treatment option for their son and acted upon it. Marketing techniques employed by proton centers help attract patients despite a dearth of substantive comparative data. Given the worldwide scarcity of access to PBT, the potential benefits of seeking PBT need to be balanced against the potential for treatment delay. This represents a common balancing act for pediatric oncologists. Luckily, despite the treatment delay, as of 2018 Ashya has returned to Southampton and is without evidence of disease.

This case perfectly encompasses the many aspects that make the cautious implementation of PBT so difficult in modern society. Often, the clinical and quality of life benefits of radiation effects cannot be measured until many years after the delivery of therapy. Late effects are truly what drive radiation dose tolerance. In a society dominated by access to information and the immediacy of social media, patients and investors are not willing to wait 10–20 years to assess the clinical benefit of a proton versus a photon. National and private health insurance companies, however, are not willing to pay for potential or theoretical benefits of therapy as these perceived benefits are often overly optimistic.

The Challenge of Cost Containment and Evidence-Based Medicine

In an era of cost containment in medicine and value-based care, PBT faces obvious scrutiny. With increasing demands for evidence-based medicine from payers, comparative data often is required to support the use of a more expensive technology. This has been the case for IMRT over conventional radiation therapy for decades, as it is the more expensive modality. Proponents of PBT argue that randomized prospective data is not necessary to prove the benefit of PBT as there is lack of equipoise given the clear improvement in dose distribution to normal tissues. Some have posited that were PBT cheaper than photon therapy, there would be no interest in performing clinical trials to substantiate their utility. A recent study showed that phase III comparative trials account for only 9% of proton clinical trials and that there has been a downtrend in PBT trials over the past 5 years despite continued development of proton centers [16]. PBT trials are rarely industry or nationally sponsored and are predominantly run by universities and hospitals. There is no drug company to fund them! It also is difficult to enroll patients on a randomized trial comparing the two modalities, when equal access exists to both due to patient preference. Simply put, if a patient can choose to receive PBT without randomization, they will make that choice.

Recently, the first phase III trial comparing advanced PBT and photon therapy planning for locally advanced lung cancer was reported [17]. The trial demonstrated no significant benefit of PBT over photon therapy in terms of risk for radiation pneumonitis or severe inflammation of the lung. Pneumonitis rates were higher in PBT patients (10.5% vs 6.5%). Survival and local control of the tumor were similar among the groups. This trial demonstrates that the theoretical benefit is not always realized in a clinically meaningful way, as so often is seen in medicine. The researchers were able to demonstrate a learning curve with improved outcomes for both protons and photons over time. Often, technology advances at a pace far quicker than clinical trial results can be obtained. Given that radiation delivery continues to evolve, by the time a given trial's results mature, they may no longer be clinically meaningful.

Proton Therapy Market

Marketing and reputation are the key market drivers in this competitive space. Marketing plays a huge role in attracting patients to medical centers. One analysis estimated hospital specialties will receive a 5% increase in non-emergency Medicare patients based on a single ranking improvement in US News and World Report rankings [18]. Interestingly, the US News and World Report rankings include "advanced technologies" in the scoring system for cancer center scoring. These rankings also have an impact on attracting wealthy international patients to major centers. In marketing, the *halo effect* can have significant impact on market share and profits. As proton centers are in their relative infancy, PBT provides a rare opportunity for medical centers to distinguish themselves on a national and international scale. While medical consumers may be attracted to a facility because of the existence of protons, even if a payer denies treatment or PBT is not indicated, the patient is more likely to receive treatment at that facility. At one large center, for example, approximately 25% of patients who contact the center about PBT go on to receive conventional treatment at the center. Simply having the proton technology available conveys a sense of excellence that drives the patient to travel to that center for their treatment. In these settings, it is more important to be perceived as better than to have real data to support that you are in fact better.

Market pressures have driven more sensibility into the PBT sector. Smaller facilities with only 1–2 rooms are increasingly common as they are cheaper to build and maintain and have a higher likelihood of keeping the room filled with paying patients to cover costs. With these units, cancer centers can offer PBT without relying on a patient draw larger than the local market. In New York, rather than several hospital systems competing individually for patients at great cost and financial risk, cancer treatment centers have entered a joint demonstration project, proposing a collaborative facility with substantial infrastructure to perform rigorous research on PBT efficacy. This collaborative approach will serve the New York Community in a more sensible manner by increasing the probability of a wide referral base and mitigating the risk of substantial losses.

Well-conducted research and reliable data about outcomes, coupled with a large patient experience, will help PBT find its correct place in the menu of cancer treatment options available to cancer patients. Collaborative programs such as that being explored in New York will help to establish the proton niche where PBT can provide a real advantage over complex photon therapy for select patients. Securing the long-term future of this emerging technology will ensure that those patients who will benefit from PBT will receive it and those who can benefit from other less expensive photon-based therapies will not be lured into unneeded higher cost PBT. In short, restoring sense and sensibility to decision-making in beam-based cancer treatment will benefit both the patient population and the market.

References

1. Wilson RR. Radiological use of fast protons. Radiology. 1946;47(5):487–91.
2. Zietman AL. Particle therapy at the "tipping point": an introduction to the Red Journal's Special Edition. Int J Radiat Oncol Biol Phys. 2016;95(1):1–3.
3. Dalwadi SM, Szeja SS, Bernicker EH, Butler EB, Teh BS, Farach AM. Practice patterns and outcomes in elderly stage I non-small cell lung cancer: a 2004-2012 SEER analysis. Clin Lung Cancer. 2018;19(2):e269–76.
4. Hancock J. As proton centers struggle, a sign of a health care bubble? Kaiser Health News, May 2, 2018. https://khn.org/news/as-proton-centers-struggle-a-sign-of-a-health-care-bubble/.
5. Hansen Z. Proton beams zap cancer with muni-bonds as market strains. Bloomberg March 13, 2018. https://www.bloomberg.com/news/articles/2018-03-13/proton-beams-zap-cancer-with-muni-bond-cash-as-market-strains.
6. Langreth R. Prostate cancer therapy too good to be true explodes health cost. Bloomberg March 25, 2012. https://www.bloomberg.com/news/articles/2012-03-26/prostate-cancer-therapy-too-good-to-be-true-explodes-health-cost.
7. Kupelian P, Kuban D, Thames H, Levy L, Horwitz E, Martinez A, Michalski J, Pisansky T, Sandler H, Shipley W, Zelefsky M, Zietman A. Improved biochemical relapse-free survival with increased external radiation doses in patients with localized prostate cancer: the combined experience of nine institutions in patients treated in 1994 and 1995. Int J Radiat Oncol Biol Phys. 2005;61(2):415–9.
8. Michalski JM, Yan Y, Watkins-Bruner D, Bosch W, Winter K, Galvin JM, Bahary J-P, Morton GC, Parliament MB, Sandler HM. Preliminary toxicity analysis of 3DCRT versus IMRT on the high dose arm of the RTOG 0126 prostate cancer trial. Int J Radiat Oncol Biol Phys. 2013;87(5):932–8.
9. Zietman AL, DeSilvio ML, Slater JD, Rossi CJ Jr, Miller DW, Adams JA, Shipley WU. Comparison of conventional-dose vs high-dose conformal radiation therapy in clini-

cally localized adenocarcinoma of the prostate: a randomized controlled trial. JAMA. 2005;294(10):1233–9.

10. Yu JB, Soulos PR, Herrin J, Cramer LD, Potosky AL, Roberts KB, Gross CP. Proton versus intensity-modulated radiotherapy for prostate cancer: patterns of care and early toxicity. J Nathl Cancer Inst. 2013;105(1):25–32.

11. Proton Beam Therapy for Prostate Cancer. Molina Healthcare, 2016. http://www.molina-healthcare.com/providers/wa/medicaid/resource/PDF/MCG-153-Proton-Beam-Therapy-for-Prostate-Cancer.pdf.

12. Proton Beam Therapy, ASTRO Model Policies, 2013 https://www.astro.org/uploaded-Files/_MAIN_SITE/Daily_Practice/Reimbursement/Model_Policies/Content_Pieces/ASTROPBTModelPolicy.pdf.

13. National Proton Beam Therapy Service Development Programme: the strategic outline case and accompanying value for money addendum. United Kingdom Department of Health and Social Care Oct 12, 2012. https://www.gov.uk/government/publications/national-proton-beam-therapy-service-development-programme.

14. Lannering B, Rutkowski S, Doz F, Pizer B, Gustafsson G, Navajas A, Massimino M, Reddingius R, Benesch M, Carrie C, Taylor R, Gandola L, Björk-Eriksson T, Giralt J, Oldenburger F, Pietsch T, Figarella-Branger D, Robson K, Forni M, Clifford SC, Warmuth-Metz M, von Hoff K, Faldum A, Mosseri V, Kortmann R. Hyperfractionated versus conventional radiotherapy followed by chemotherapy in standard-risk medulloblastoma: results from the randomized multicenter HIT-SIOP PNET 4 trial. J Clin Oncol. 2012;30(26):3187–93.

15. Yock TI, Yeap BY, Ebb DH, Weyman E, Eaton BR, Sherry NA, Jones RM, MacDonald SM, Pulsifer MB, Lavally B, Abrams AN, Huang MS, Marcus KJ, Tarbell NJ. Long-term toxic effects of proton radiotherapy for paediatric medulloblastoma: a phase 2 single-arm study. Lancet Oncol. 2016;17(3):287–98.

16. Odei BCL, Boothe D, Keole SR, Vargas CE, Foote RL, Schild SE, Ashman JB. A 20-year analysis of clinical trials involving proton beam therapy. Int J Particle Ther Winter. 2016;3(3):398–406.

17. Liao Z, Lee JJ, Komaki R, Gomez DR, O'Reilly MS, Fossella FV, Blumenschein GR, Heymach JV, Vaporciyan AA, Swisher SG, Allen PK, Choi NC, DeLaney TF, Hahn SM, Cox JD, Lu CS, Mohan R. Bayesian adaptive randomization trial of passive scattering proton therapy and intensity-modulated photon radiotherapy for locally advanced non–small-cell lung cancer. J Clin Oncol. 2018;36(18):1813–22.

18. Pope DG. Reacting to rankings: evidence from "America's Best Hospitals". J Health Economics. 2009;28:1154–65.

Chapter 11
The Ethics of Animal Use in Cancer Research

Bernard E. Rollin

Introduction: Conceptual and Ethical Background

The relationship between science and society is not a warm one – at best it is like a bad marriage. If one asks the scientists they will, with some justification, cite societal ignorance of basic science as a good reason to dismiss social concern about science's activities, including animal research. The general public in the United States is indeed extraordinarily ignorant, in a know-nothing, aggressive way, regarding basic principles of science in all areas. Thus, for example, it has been pointed out by a prominent scholar of scientific literacy that the United States consistently ranks low compared to other developed countries on assessments of scientific literacy and that "recent international comparisons have shown that approximately one in four American adults qualifies as scientifically literate" [7]. Miller also points out that "only 28 percent of American adults have sufficient understanding of basic scientific ideas to be able to read the Science section in the Tuesday *New York Times*" (Ibid.).

In a 2004 paper, neuroscientist and physician Dr. Keith Black affirmed that research shows that "One half of the American public does not know the earth goes around the sun once a year…. A 1996 National Assessment Educational Progress survey found that 43 percent of high school seniors did not meet the basic standard for scientific knowledge" [1]. A 2016 Pew Charitable Trusts report on scientific literacy indicates that 40% of the US public believe that humans coexisted with the dinosaurs (Pew 2016). And a 2015 survey showed that 80% of the public wanted mandatory labeling of food indicating the presence of DNA [17].

B. E. Rollin (✉)
Philosophy, Colorado State University, Fort Collins, CO, USA
e-mail: Bernard.Rollin@Colostate.edu

© Springer Nature Switzerland AG 2019
E. H. Bernicker (ed.), *Cancer and Society*,
https://doi.org/10.1007/978-3-030-05855-5_11

A 2014 Gallup poll cited in a National Center for Science Education report stated that only a very small percentage (19%) of the US public has accepted the naturalistic position that "man has developed over millions of years from less advanced forms of life. God had no part in this process" [9] (http://www.gallup.com/poll/21814/Evolution-Creationism-Intelligent-Design.aspx). Correlatively, a 2017 Gallup poll indicated that "the percentage of Americans who actively want creation not evolution to be taught in schools may seem relatively modest at 30%, but this number is significantly larger than the percentage who actively want evolution to be taught over creation" [5].

Beginning in the 1960s and continuing through the present, science has become something of a political football for both the political left and the political right. For the left, objectivity is allegedly a myth perpetuated by the ruling class, and the attack on objectivity has taken the form of radical relativism and subjectivism. The best articulation of this position can be found in philosopher of science Paul Feyerabend's *Science in a Free Society*, specifically arguing that the hegemony of science is expressly anti-democratic [3]. For example, Feyerabend has affirmed that putting scientists rather than Navajo shamans on national policy committees represents a salient example. For the right, scientific thinking is a cudgel for attacking traditional values and traditional beliefs and threatens to erode parental authority.

Awareness of this unfortunate state is nothing new. In 1964, Richard Hofstadter's monumental historical study, *Anti-Intellectualism in American Life,* won the Pulitzer Prize for chronicling the ubiquitous anti-intellectual posture that is a major and dominant strain in American thought [6]. Less than a decade earlier, British scholar C. P. Snow bemoaned the huge academic chasm that separated scientists from scholars in the arts and humanities. And not only is the United States anti-intellectual, we are openly hostile to science. As Jeffrey Sachs wrote in *The Economist,* September 22, 2008: "By anti-intellectualism I mean an aggressively anti-scientific perspective, backed by disdain for those who adhere to science and evidence" [16].

By the same token, on the other side, science has done little to address societal ignorance. Furthermore, science has been captured by an ideological framework so ubiquitous that I have called it "the common sense of science," for it is to scientists what ordinary common sense is to daily life [13].

This ideology encompasses two components directly relevant to the topic at hand. The first component is the ubiquitous denial of the relevance or even presence of ethics in science. This claim is readily evidenced in the failure of science textbooks, for example, biology texts, to articulate ethical issues occasioned by science. There are ubiquitous claims in what my colleague calls "the throat-clearing introduction" to standard textbooks affirming that "science is value- free" in general and "ethics-free" in particular. The standard line was that science supplies good information on the basis of which *society* can make ethical decisions but does not itself make ethical judgments. The claim was based in the simplistic view that science deals only with *what is empirically observable or testable*, and as Wittgenstein remarked, if one inventories all the facts in the universe, one does not find it a fact that killing is wrong [18].

The most dramatic (and chilling) encapsulation of this ideology can be found in a statement made by the director of NIH, which position, it is important to remember, requires both excellent scientific abilities and political astuteness. In 1989, the then director of NIH and therefore arguably the chief representative of biomedicine in the United States was visiting his alma mater. He was talking to a group of students informally, and was apparently unguarded in his remarks, not realizing that a student reporter for the school paper was present. The students asked him about the ethical issues associated with genetic engineering. His reply was astonishing: He opined that "though scientific advances like genetic engineering are always controversial, *science should never be hampered by ethical considerations*" [8]. When I pose the question to my students of who made that statement in the twentieth century, they invariably say "Hitler."

The second ideological dogma I encountered was a ubiquitous belief that scientists needed to be agnostic about animal thought and feeling, and even about animal pain, since one could not verify claims about animal mentation empirically. Interestingly enough, Darwin himself took for granted the fact that if physiological and metabolic traits were phylogenetically continuous, so too were mental traits, and he wrote extensively about them, for an example in his *Expression of the Emotions in Man and Animals* [2], and even did empirical research on the problem-solving abilities of earthworms! And although modern biology claims to be solidly Darwinian, by 1920 virtually no one in biology or psychology accepted the existence of thought and feelings in animals. (See [12] for detailed discussion.)

It was in good measure the moral imperative to introduce pain control into science that led my colleagues and I to draft what became the 1985 Amendments to the Animal Welfare Act requiring control of any research modalities causing pain and distress in animals in the course of research. Though the research community protested that they used copious amounts of analgesia, a literature search I performed in 1982 through the Library of Congress *was unable to find a single paper dealing with "analgesia for laboratory animals."* This was instrumental in convincing the Congress of the necessity for such legislation. Until the passage of the law, which went into effect in 1987, there was virtually no analgesia used by the research community, nor was it deployed or taught in veterinary schools or veterinary practices. In fact, with the exception of one cream applied to cattle hooves for cases of "foot rot," a very painful bacterial infection, *there are still no analgesics approved for any use in food animals!*

The conditions just described – social ignorance about science coupled with scientific agnosticism about ethics and feelings in animals – inexorably led to a perfect storm with both sides consistently talking past each other. The situation created what I have elsewhere called a "Gresham's law for ethics." It will be recalled that Gresham's law affirms that bad money (e.g., the worthless paper money circulating in post-World War I Germany) drives good money out of circulation. In the same way, "bad ethics drives good ethics out of circulation." When preparing to address the Congress on animal research, I performed a literature search for scientific papers addressing the ethics of animal research and found nothing. By the same token, given public ignorance of science and lack of sophistication in ethics, issues were defined by alarmists, theologians, and others to whom ethics was essentially emotion. A superb example of this is provided by a survey conducted by Time Warner after the announcement of a research group having created a cloned animal, Dolly the sheep. In response to queries about the ethics of cloning, fully three out of four Americans declared that the cloning of Dolly "violated God's will."

Implications of the Tension Between Science and Society

This fairly detailed introduction is essential in order to understand the debate about the ethics of animal research. The major point to stress is that the general public clearly sees the invasive use of animals in research as a moral issue, and about 50% disapprove of such use [10]. Given the point made earlier that the same public is often unclear about what are legitimate ethical issues as opposed to spurious ones – witness the Dolly case just enumerated – it seems obvious that the burden is on the research community to, in a fair way, delineate the ethical issues occasioned by animal research and their rational response to these issues. This is because, as the president of a major European swine company indicated, the general public is in a position to determine the playing field upon which animal use, be it agriculture or research, is played out.

For example, during the early 1980s, I was party to an Australian parliamentary discussion, led by a prominent Senator, that was seriously considering creating a legislative ban on animal research in Australia! In the same vein, in the mid-1980s, there was a serious bill supported by animal activists in the United States that would have cut the federal animal research budget by up to 60% and devoted the money to alternatives to animal use.

For most of Western history, the societal consensus ethic for animals, i.e., what was codified in law, was extremely minimalistic. In antiquity, when most animal use was agricultural and based in husbandry, self-interest assured good animal treatment. Inflicting unnecessary or sadistic suffering on animals was condemned in biblical teaching and explicitly attacked by St. Thomas Aquinas on the basis of the psychological insight that those who abuse animals will graduate to abusing people, an insight that has been solidly supported by twentieth century psychology and psychiatry. The prohibition against deliberate cruelty was encoded in the laws of all civilized societies beginning in the late eighteenth century in Britain.

By the second half of the twentieth century, society became well aware of the fact that most animal suffering was not the result of deliberate, sadistic cruelty of the sort condemned by the anti-cruelty ethic. In fact, the vast majority of animal suffering was understood to be the result of normal, decent motivations such as providing cheap and plentiful food, advancing scientific knowledge, and assuring the safety of consumer products. During the ensuing years, it has become ever-increasingly evident to society in general that the law is a powerful tool for raising the status of animals.

Thus, for example, in 2004, there were 2100 pieces of legislation floated in federal, state, and local legislatures in the United States aimed at enhancing the welfare of animals. The societal thrust has continued to grow. In 2003, a Gallup poll indicated that approximately 70% of the US public wished to see legislated constraints on how farm animals could be raised (Gallup 2003). When the survey was recently repeated in 2012, the number had risen to 94% (Gallup 2012). This point is further buttressed by referenda aimed at limiting the most egregious confinement of farm animals – veal crates, sow stalls, and battery cages for chickens. In each of 12 states that the referendum was floated, it passed by a 2 to 1 margin. A recent speech by the executive director of the Foundation for Biomedical Research, perhaps the major lobby group for biomedicine, rightly stressed that animal advocacy had shifted from radical action to attempting to change public policy.

Other signs of increased concern with animal welfare are manifest across the world. California banned killer whale shows. Ringling Brothers Circus has closed after more than 100 years of popularity. Zoos as essentially prisons for animals have disappeared. Spain has experienced major protests against bullfighting. The practice of cutting off fins from sharks and then throwing the animals back is being vehemently attacked.

What do we know about societal ethics regarding animal research? One obvious point is that society does not wish animals to suffer pain or distress. Connected with this, and particularly evident with regard to farm animals, is that social ethics wants to see animals' basic needs as determined by their biological and psychological natures respected. This claim is supported by the worldwide rejection of extreme confinement systems for farm animals, as indicated earlier. In my own experience, I was able in 2008 to convince Smithfield Farms, the largest pork producer in America, to abandon gestation crates after I advised them to poll their customers, and they subsequently found that 78% of those customers despised such crates. Battery cages for laying hens are being abandoned, and egg companies trumpet that they produce cage-free eggs. Veal crates are gone, with veal calves being raised in groups.

On the other hand, it is also evident in the food animal area that members of the public do not worry about the fact that animals are killed to be eaten. What they do worry about is not *that* they are killed but *how* they are killed, i.e., without pain, distress, and fear. Hence the major emphasis is placed on stunning of food animals in the beef industry to assure that they are rendered unconscious instantaneously, statistically most often by the use of a "captive bolt pistol" that, if placed properly, eventuates in immediate loss of awareness. Unfortunately, stunning in the pork and chicken industries is far less effective, and one might argue is horrendously unacceptable in what the animal experiences before being killed. But for our purposes, the key point is that the social ethic does not worry about the fact of animal death but rather about how it is accomplished. Significant portions of northern Europe have correlatively banned kosher and halal slaughter, accomplished by cutting the throat of a conscious animal.

The obvious question that arises is why this is the case? How do animals value death as compared with pain and suffering? This in turn leads to an ancillary question – can an animal value life per se? To answer this question, we must consider some conceptual differences between animal and human cognition.

Human cognition is such that we can value long-term future goals and endure short-run negative experiences for the sake of achieving them. Examples are plentiful. Many of us undergo voluntary food restriction, and the unpleasant experience attendant in its wake, for the sake of lowering blood pressure or looking good in a bathing suit as summer approaches. We memorize volumes of boring material for the sake of gaining admission to veterinary or medical school. We endure the excruciating pain of cosmetic surgery to look better.

In the case of animals, however, there is no evidence, either empirical or conceptual, that they have the capability to weigh future benefits or possibilities against current misery. To entertain the belief that "my current pain and distress, resulting from the nausea of chemotherapy or some highly invasive surgery, will be offset by the possibility of an indefinite amount of future time" is taken to be axiomatic of human thinking. But reflection reveals that such thinking requires some complex cognitive machinery. For example, one needs temporal and abstract concepts, such as possible future times and the ability to compare them, and a concept of death, eloquently defined by Heidegger as "grasping the possibility of the impossibility of your being." It is also equally evident that an animal cannot weigh being treated for cancer against the suffering treatment entails, cannot affirm a desire (or even conceive of a desire) to endure current suffering for the sake of future life, and cannot understand that current suffering may be counterbalanced by future life.

A very important corollary emerges from our discussion. We have argued that animals have no concept of death (or life) and consequently cannot value it more than pain. We have also indicated that people sometimes value death over pain, as a way of ending pain. If this is true of humans, it would be a fortiori true of animals, who cannot value life at all. Thus, in a sense, pain may well be worse for animals than for humans, as they cannot rationalize its acceptance by appeal to future life without pain. As I have said in other writings, a traditional argument affirms that human pain is worse than animal pain because humans can anticipate and fear pain very imaginatively before it happens, as when we plan to visit the dentist. Aside from the fact that animals too can fear *imminent* pain (e.g., when they cringe before a threatening upraised hand), the same logic decrees that animals cannot look forward to a time without the pain; their entire universe is the pain, and they can have no *hope*!

None of this is to suggest that society would be cavalier about taking animal life. Noteworthy in this regard is a survey performed by *Glamour* magazine in the 1970s. Amazingly enough, even though one can assume that the readership of *Glamour* was strongly biased toward new cosmetics, the majority of their readership indicated that making animals suffer was not justified by new products! During the ensuing years, a large number of cosmetics companies have gone on to disavow animal testing, beginning with the Body Shoppe. In other words, even people with a vested interest in a certain sort of animal testing will distinguish between testing that is worthwhile in regard to taking an animal's life and making the animal suffer and testing that is not warranted. As we have already mentioned, according to a 2015 Pew report, a full 50% of Americans disapprove of the practice of testing on animals, regardless of the purpose to which the testing is put, up from 26% in 2001.

(In the interest of fairness, I must say that I take polls with a grain of salt, though they are doubtless good general indicators.)

All of this explains the spectacular success of the Center for Alternatives to Animal Testing developed at Johns Hopkins some 40 years ago, as well as the proliferation of cellular and molecular alternatives to animal use. As I write this in February 2018, there is a bill before the Congress entitled HR 2790, the Humane Cosmetics Act, designed to end the use of animals for safety testing of cosmetics. Research on chimpanzees has been stopped by NIH.

Cosmetic testing is not the only use of animals in science perceived as unacceptable by large portions of society. Many people also feel that diseases arising from lifestyle choices such as smoking, which are viewed as "self-inflicted," should not be studied in animals.

We can summarize the societal ethic regarding animal testing as follows: in the course of animal testing, the animals should not suffer pain or distress. Testing that is done should be done for valuable medical purposes, not frivolous ones. A significant number of people see the use of animals in research as morally wrong. Animal research should promise specific and tangible human benefits. Animals used in research should be kept under conditions that accommodate their biological and psychological natures. (Not only is this an ethical imperative; it is also a scientific one. Failing to meet the animals' nature deforms critical physiological and metabolic variables, thereby placing the research validity in jeopardy.)

Animals in Cancer Research

What then does this tell us about the use of animals in cancer research? As common sense and our own experience tell us, there are few diseases inspiring the naked terror in people that cancer does. It thus stands to reason that animal research on cancer is likely to be the most socially acceptable use of animals, indeed more so than any other animal research modality. Such acceptability would presumably require, ideally, causing as little pain in the animals as possible and, ideally, no pain. Painless death, as we argued earlier, seems to be socially accepted. We must also recall that pain deforms relevant physiological and metabolic variables that researchers are attempting to study. Thus there is a methodological as well as a moral reason to avoid having animals used in cancer research suffer pain and distress.

In addition, veterinary epidemiology has begun to study historical and current hospital records of animals afflicted with cancer as a viable alternative to creating the disease in animals. Furthermore, veterinary animal cancer researchers are more and more using their treating of companion animals afflicted with cancer as a way of studying the disease, both in terms of etiology and treatment. Not only does this not generate public disapproval, it garners major contributions from wealthy pet owners. In 1982, *The Wall Street Journal* reported on such people spending over 100 thousand dollars on their animal's cancer treatment. Shortly thereafter, Colorado State University College of Veterinary Medicine built a cancer building with grateful donor contributions from clients and with funding from NIH. In a news report aired in February 2018, it was reported that "Humans and dogs are 95% identical genetically—and the diseases that affect humans, including breast cancer, prostate cancer, and melanoma, are almost identical." (This is not strictly true of melanomas.) In short, modalities for studying cancer in animals are emerging that create a win-win situation for humans and animals, most notably for the companion animals that over 90% of the public view as "members of the family."

What of animal use in cancer research where this happy coincidence does not obtain? In particular, what of "non-favored animals" such as rats and mice? There is absolutely no reason to believe that society is unconcerned about such animals, as we saw evidenced by the rejection of cosmetic testing. There is in fact survey data promulgated by the Humane Society of the United States showing an inverse correlation between public support for animal research and the degree of pain and suffering inflicted on animals. When one reaches a stage of creating uncontrolled suffering in research animals, public support for such research drops precipitously.

Thus it would very much behoove the cancer research community to abide by established principles for limiting animal pain and suffering. These principles include strict limits on the size of tumors that are allowed to develop in research animals. It was not that long ago that animals were allowed to develop tumors as big as they were! A related principle is to demand euthanasia of animals afflicted with cancer before symptoms that hurt the animals are allowed to develop. (In animal research, these are known as "endpoints" and are established at the beginning of the study.)

On the other hand, researchers are developing tumors in rodents that are orthotopic, i.e., develop at the actual point such tumors naturally arise, for example, in the pancreas, as opposed to being simply implanted subcutaneously. Such surgeries will require more analgesia not only during implantation, but as the tumors grow and impair normal function. More than ever, therefore, early endpoints will be required in addition to increased analgesia.

And I cannot stress enough that euthanasia should be what its name suggests – a good death for the animal, not necessarily the easiest, most convenient death as far as the researcher is concerned. In my view, for example, the standardly accepted death by CO_2 inhalation is *not* a good death; it is after all asphyxiation or suffocation, far from a good death. Whenever possible, animals should be offered for adoption at the end of a research protocol. These simple principles, coupled with the importance of cancer research, go a long way toward satisfying public moral concern.

In addition, there is voluminous scientific literature indicating that satisfying what Aristotle called an animal's *telos*, i.e., its psychological and biological nature, is of great importance to animals used in research. In fact, there is research indicating that satisfaction of the animals' natures is more important to them than pain control, as animals when caught in steel-jawed traps will chew their legs off in order to escape, evidencing the fact that freedom of movement is more important than pain [14, 15]. In addition, respecting animal natures removes the stress that ignoring it imposes upon research results from a physiological, pharmacological, and metabolic perspective. In fact, unfortunately, researchers are often quite cavalier about managing stress variables that can well deform their results. And it should never be forgotten that pain is a significant stressor.

As an excellent example, consider the following: In one research protocol with which I was personally familiar, beagles used to study mammary cancer were housed in large kennels where the barking was so loud that caretakers and researchers had to wear ear protectors, though the dogs did not. Ironically, an article had appeared in *Science* showing that beagles subjected to unmitigated stressors *such as noise* developed more mammary tumors than unstressed animals [11].

It is for this reason that when my colleagues and I drafted the 1985 Amendments to the Animal Welfare Act, we stipulated that animals should be housed and maintained in accord with their natures. Unfortunately, the Congress only approved some facsimile of this principle for dogs and nonhuman primates. For cancer researchers to adopt this principle would be a highly moral, prudential, and effective modality for solidifying public support and should assure better science.

Conclusion

An end to tension between scientific ideology on the one hand and social ethics and social lack of understanding of science is essential. Making the public scientifically literate is extremely difficult to achieve, as it would require restructuring of our educational system. Repairing scientific ideology should be somewhat easier but is by no means simple. For over 40 years, I have been urging the scientific community to incorporate ethical education into the science curricula at all levels. The response from NIH and NSF has been to mandate the teaching of what a barbarous neologism calls "regulatory compliance." For example, there is a new 500-page series of edicts pertaining to human research that is essentially just a list of rules. Far more efficacious would be the teaching of genuine ethics as an integral part of teaching science, particularly the life sciences and biomedical science.

A colleague and I taught a freshman 1 year of honors biology class for over 20 years where ethics was part and parcel of the curriculum. The results far exceeded our expectations. I still occasionally receive letters of thanks from students who went through the course and realize how much more comprehension they have of the place of science in society and the role of ethics in science. I have also taught a graduate course in science and ethics for 15 years with similar results. As Plato pointed out long ago, having good people in society is far superior to having good laws. And as Plato also pointed out, the surest mechanism for creating good people is providing good education. This is particularly true regarding the socio-ethical playing field upon which science occurs.

Acknowledgment I am grateful to Dr. Daniel Gustafson for incisive comments on an earlier version of this manuscript and for extremely helpful dialogue. I am also grateful to Dr. Terry Engle for his comments on the manuscript.

References

1. Black K. Scientific illiteracy in the U.S. Cedars-Sinai neurosciences report; 2004.
2. Darwin C. The expression of the emotions in man and animals. New York: Greenwood; 1872/1969.
3. Feyerabend P. Science in a free society. New York: Verso Books; 1978.
4. Gallup polls.: http://www.Gallup.com.
5. Gallup. 2017. news.gallup.com/poll/16462/americans-weigh-evolution-vs-creationism-schools. aspx.
6. Hofstadter R. Anti-intellectualism in American life. New York: Knopf; 1963.
7. Miller J. Chapter 12. The conceptualization and measurement of civic scientific literacy for the twenty-first century. In: Meinwald J, Hildebrand JG, editors. Science and the educated American: a core component of liberal education. Cambridge, MA: American Academy of Arts and Sciences; 2010.. https://www.amacad.org/content/publications/pubContent.aspx?d=1118.
8. Michigan State News, February 27, 1989.
9. National Center for Science Education. 2014. Opinion about the use of animals in research. https://ncse.com/news/2014/06/latest-gallup-poll-evolution-0015653.
10. Pew Research Center. September 10, 2015. A look at what the public knows and does not know about science. http://www.pewinternet.org/2015/09/10/what-the-public-knows-and-does-not-know-about-science/.
11. Riley V. Mouse mammary tumors: alteration of incidence as apparent function of stress. Science. 1975;189(4201):465–7.
12. Rollin B. The unheeded cry: animal consciousness, animal pain and science. New York: Oxford University Press; 1989.
13. Rollin B. Science and ethics. New York: Cambridge University Press; 2007.
14. Rollin B. Beyond pain – controlling suffering in laboratory animals. Bioscience. 2015;65(12):1113–4.
15. Rollin B. A new basis for animal ethics – telos and common sense. Columbia: University of Missouri Press; 2016.
16. Sachs J. The American anti-intellectual threat. Business World; September 25, 2008.
17. Washington Post. January 17, 2015. Over 80% of Americans support "mandatory labels on food containing DNA".
18. Wittgenstein L. Lecture on ethics. Philos Rev. 1965;74(1):3–12.

Chapter 12
The Ecology of Cancer

Beata Ujvari, Jay Fitzpatrick, Nynke Raven, Jens Osterkamp, and Frédéric Thomas

Introduction

It is now widely established that multicellular organisms are not autonomous entities, but rather "holobionts" composed of the host plus all of its commensal and mutualistic microorganisms, as well as a diversity of pathogens/parasites (viruses, bacteria, fungi, protozoa and metazoans) [1]. Extensive research has unambiguously shown the significant impact of pathogens/parasites on the host phenotype [2]. These studies have also demonstrated that the eco-evolutionary dynamics of animals (hosts) and symbionts (encompassing all types of symbioses) are inextricably linked [2]. In addition to microbiota and pathogens/parasites, multicellular organisms "host" a third category of symbiont: the community of altered "selfish" cells, malignant cells (oncobiota) [3]. Malignant cells originate from normal cells that abandon their cooperative behaviour, become neoplastic, proliferate at greater rates than somatic cells and disseminate throughout the body. Cancer is an ancient phenomenon that is linked to the appearance and evolution of multicellular organisms (metazoans) [4, 5]. Transitioning from an unicellular life form to multicellularity required the sophisticated, higher-level cooperation of cells with complementary behaviours (reviewed in [5, 6]). The emergence of genes facilitating cell

B. Ujvari (✉) · J. Fitzpatrick · N. Raven
Centre for Integrative Ecology, School of Life and Environmental Sciences,
Deakin University, Geelong, Waurn Ponds, VIC, Australia
e-mail: beata.ujvari@deakin.edu.au

J. Osterkamp
Department of Surgery and Transplantation, Rigshospitalet, Copenhagen Ø,
Denmark

F. Thomas
CREEC, Montpellier, France

MIVEGEC, UMR IRD/CNRS/UM 5290, Montpellier, France

© Springer Nature Switzerland AG 2019
E. H. Bernicker (ed.), *Cancer and Society*,
https://doi.org/10.1007/978-3-030-05855-5_12

cooperation resulted in the evolution of stable multicellularity [4]. However, optimal functioning of multicellular organisms requires strict regulation of overall cell proliferation levels and cell numbers [7] and a constant control of neoplastic cells [7]. When the balance is broken, neoplastic cells that acquire genetic and/or epigenetic mutations conferring higher fitness (growth advantage and/or proliferative potential) are selected and expanded, ensued by oncogenesis and neoplasm/tumour formation [8, 9]. Neoplasms are composed of an admixture of clones that not only compete for resources but also cooperate to avoid immune recognition and are thus able to disperse and colonize new organs. Intra-tumour genetic, epigenetic and phenotypic heterogeneity provides the evolutionary landscape for individual cancer cells to adapt to selection pressures imposed by the microenvironment (immune system and other tumour suppression mechanisms). Cancer cells are able to rapidly acquire novel phenotypes: immortalization, invasiveness and resistance [10, 11]. Except for transmissible cancers (see [12]), cancer development and progression are evolutionary processes within a single host where the host's immune system selects for malignant cells that are resistance to immune attacks and can transmit to novel organs [10, 11, 13, 14]. However, the ultimate fate of malignant cells is to expire with the death of the host organism, as the breakdown of cellular cooperation leads to metastatic cancer and ultimately to the death of multicellular organisms [6].

Neoplasia, being the disease of multicellular organisms, is indeed not only a major cause of human death worldwide that touches nearly every family on the planet but has also been recorded in numerous invertebrate [15, 16] and vertebrate [17–19] species (reviewed in [20]). Similar to other diseases, cancer is a significant physiological burden on the host [21–23] and hence alters the behaviour of individuals and impacts interindividual interactions. It has been proposed that cancer may have a significant ecological impact on trophic cascades, niche allocation, host-parasite dynamics and disease epidemiology of the ecosystem occupied by the affected host species [12].

In this chapter we provide an overview of the ecology of cancer at the scale of micro- (host) and macro-ecosystems (species). We discuss the underlying mechanisms driving malignant and metastatic formations in the tissue environment and then investigate the impact of neoplasia on individuals, species and populations. Finally, we provide suggestions on how understanding the ecology of cancer can contribute to both cancer prevention and development of new treatment strategies.

The Ecology of Cancer at the Micro-Ecosystem Scale

A cancer cell's fitness is governed by its own proliferation rate, thus cells that maximize proliferation in local tissues, followed by transmission to novel organs (once resources are depleted at the site of initiation) will have higher fitness compared to cells with lower proliferation rates. The complex, multistep biological process of metastasis [24, 25] involves the initiation and growth of cancer cells at primary tumour sites, angiogenesis to support the developing tumour and invasion of the stromal tissue surrounding the malignant cells [26]. Once resources become limited at the site of initiation, malignant cells disassemble the extracellular matrix, enter the lymphatic or blood microvessels (intravasation) and disseminate throughout the body of the host. The vast majority of circulating tumour cells die in transit but a few survive by arresting in the capillary beds within distant organs and finally extravasate into the new host tissue [26, 27]. Invading cancer cells face an uncertain future, and some form microscopic metastases and progress no further, while a very small minority of metastatic cells form clinically apparent tumours [26].

Although the invasive metastatic cascade plays out during the lifetime of an individual, a strong analogy can be drawn from the effects of invasive species on whole ecosystems [28]. We therefore investigate the ecological basis of cancers by drawing on the analogy of invasive species colonizing novel habitats/ecosystems.

The Characteristics of Successful Invaders

The seminal works by Ehrlich [28] and Lodge [29] proposed a list of attributes of invasive species in order to successfully colonize novel areas, including (1) plastic life history strategies, (2) polyphagous (i.e. wide feeding niche), (3) abundance in their original range, (4) high genetic variability, (5) asexual and/or single-parent reproduction, (6) phenotypic plasticity and (7) ability to function in a wide range of physical conditions (reviewed in [30, 31]). Some of these attributes are directly applicable to the transitioning of primary tumour cells to metastatic invasive cells.

Plastic Life History Strategies

Similar to invasive species [32], plastic life history strategies are also relevant to the complex ecosystem of tumours, neoplastic cells showing phenotypes with fast and/or slow life history characteristics [33] and more importantly the plasticity to shift along the spectrum of different life histories to suit the environment (reviewed in [13]). Selective pressure caused by unstable microenvironment at tumour initiation sites will allow some mutant subclones with fast life history hallmarks (enhanced cell proliferating capacity, sustained proliferating signals, growth suppression evasion) to expand. However, to avoid recognition and destruction by the immune system and to overcome novel challenging conditions (such as resource-limiting environments due to limits of oxygen diffusion from the existing capillary network) may necessitate a shift towards to a slower life history strategy and hence investment into increased survival (slow life history hallmark [13]). However, the formation of new blood vessels (angiogenesis) allows cells to overcome the constraint of limited resources and to rapidly shift to a fast life history strategy. Metastasis, neoplastic cells escaping final resource limitations by invading novel micro- (within the same host) and macro-environments (invading a novel host, i.e. contagious cancers

[12]), represents fast life history strategies analogous to those observed in invasive species. Hence, successful neoplastic cells, like successful invasive species, should have the capacity to switch between fast and slow life history strategies.

Phenotypic Plasticity

Invasion is a dynamic process; in order to successfully colonize a novel environment, one or more specimens of a species or a cancer cell line must leave the original colony, survive migration and establish an initial population at the novel site, followed by colonization of larger areas [34]. Since colonists must be able to cope with a range of environmental conditions, phenotypic plasticity (change in phenotypic expression in response to environmental variations) has been singled out as one of the key life history traits needed to successful colonization of novel areas [30]. Initially only a few individuals (see propagule pressure below) of an invasive species or cells arrive to a novel area (being a novel geographic area, organ or host) and hence the colonists generally display low genetic variability (clonal selection in cancer cells). Therefore increased phenotypic plasticity may enable colonizing species/cells to cope with and become established under challenging novel environmental conditions [35]. Furthermore, phenotypic adaptations arising from a stable genetic background may enable the colonizing organism/cells to take advantage of environmental fluctuations and to outcompete the native, non-invasive species/cells at the site of colonization [36]. Phenotypic plasticity, generated by epigenetic modifications, has indeed been proposed to underlie efficient metastatic processes [24, 37–39] and the success of invasive species [40]. Epigenetic variation regulating complex gene expression signatures superimposed over the primary tumour genotype allows the invasive cancer genomes to respond to developmental and environmental cues [39, 41]. Epigenetic regulators, including DNA methylation, histone and chromatin modifications and miRNA regulation, orchestrate dynamic, adaptive and reversible phenotypic differences [42] ensuring easy transition between fast and slow life history strategies of colonizing cells. For example, cues of resource abundance could initiate a proliferative phenotype by facilitating expression of oncogenes via removing methyl groups from their promoter regions (hypomethylation) and blocking tumour suppressor genes by adding methyl groups (hypermethylation) to corresponding promoters. Once resources are scarce, by switching on the cell cycle inhibitor gene promoters and turning off pro-apoptotic genes via modulating their epigenetic state, a quiescent, dormant phenotype can be achieved [13].

Phenotypic plasticity and regulatory mechanisms are also essential to facilitate the observed bidirectional communication between cancer cells and their microenvironment [43]. Tumour cells are continuously adapting to circumvent the normalizing cues of the microenvironment, and in turn, the microenvironment evolves to accommodate the malignant cells [44]. The gene expression changes in both stromal and tumour epithelial cells result in dynamic paracrine and autocrine signalling driving tumour-stromal cell interactions as tumours evolve [45–49], demonstrating that the tumour microenvironment actively contributes to tumour initiation and supports carcinogenesis, progression and metastasis [44].

Competitiveness and Dominating the Community

Invaders employ different mechanisms to outcompete and to dominate the colonized community, for example, by releasing biochemical and secondary metabolites, invasive plants can influence growth, survival and reproduction of native species and the ecophysiological attributes of the native biota (allelopathy) [50]. Ecological facilitation and allelopathy leads to reduced competition from native species and relaxed predation pressure [31]. Similarly cancer cells often alter their microenvironment to create novel niches less favourable to competitors and to reduce the risk of predation by the immune system [51]. For example, variations in the tumour vascular network and associated blood flow, substrate and metabolite availability (such as oxygen and acid, respectively) serve as selection forces in tumour ecosystems [51].

Furthermore, cancer cells use aerobic glycolysis, or fermentation of glucose to lactic acid in the presence of oxygen ("Warburg effect" [52]), to produce energy. The result of this abnormal glycolysis is high lactic acid production and the creation of a hostile hypoxic and acidic microenvironment. Why cancer cells use such an inefficient and hazardous way of energy production (aerobic glycolysis is 18-fold less effective than oxidative phosphorylation for generating ATP) is intriguing [53, 54] and enticed various explanations [54–56]. According to the high-energy view, aerobic glycolysis enables rapidly dividing cancer cells to harness additional ATP while also generating essential biosynthetic building blocks (nucleic acid, amino acids, lipids, etc.) [54]. A population biology-based model proposes that aerobic glycolysis may confer a selective advantage in the competition for shared energy resources [57], while the tumour ecosystem approach suggests that it is a defence adaptation protecting cancer cells from the generated higher than usual oxidative and acid-induced toxic microenvironment [58]. Alternatively, aerobic glycolysis could be selected via bet-hedging as it permits malignant cells to cope with environmental fluctuations such as variation in oxygen levels [59, 60]. Due to low perfusion and highly proliferating cancer cells producing excess lactic acid, protons start accumulating at the tumour site. To maintain intracellular pH, cancer cells extrude the accumulated acid via the increased activity of several proton transporters, resulting in a normal or slightly alkaline intracellular pH, and the acidification of the extracellular microenvironment [61]. The generated acidic environment reduces the viability and function of normal cells, including immune cells, concomitantly protecting the cancer cells from the immune system. Furthermore, hypoxia and/or the acidophilic environment also supports stromal remodelling, growth of blood vessels and the escape of immune surveillance by recruiting myeloid-derived suppressor cells [62, 63]. In addition, producing ATP at a higher rate but lower yield provides malignant cells with other selective advantages such as the inducement of oncogenes by lactate, the by-product of anaerobic glycolysis [54]. Clearly, the complex allopathic interactions of tumour and microenvironment resulting in reversed intra-extracellular pH gradients and immune system evasion facilitate cancer cells to outcompete normal cells, avoid predation, proliferate and survive in a hostile environment [64–66].

Propagule Pressure

Introduction effort (propagule pressure) is one of the key factors exerting strong controlling influences on invasion processes [67]. Therefore the probability of a successful colonization depends on (i) the number of propagules/cells released, (ii) the number of introduction attempts and rate and (iii) temporal and spatial patterns of propagule arrival (including proximity to existing populations of invaders) (reviewed in [34, 67, 68]). Demographic and environmental stochasticity may reduce establishment success; however increasing the propagule size and the number of invasion events can diminish the negative impact of such demographic and environmental processes. Furthermore, ongoing propagule pressure may increase genetic variation and hence overcomes the potential negative effect of bottleneck initiated by the invasion of low numbers of individuals/cells [34].

Micro-Ecosystem Attributes Facilitating Cell Invasion

Apart from the characteristics of invasive species and cancer cells facilitating progression and invasion, incursion success also depends on the invasibility of the colonized area [69]. Disturbed environments have been shown to be subjected to significantly more invasive species compared to pristine habitats [51, 70]. Thus, while cancer site invasibility likely depends primarily on immune privileged status and on the host's immune competence [71], inflamed, infected or injured tissues or hosts may be more permissive for cancer cell growth and establishment [70]. Chronic irritation, inflammation and infections are critical components of tumour emergence and progression. Inflammatory cells orchestrate the tumour microenvironment and foster neoplastic cell proliferation, survival and migration. Additionally malignant cells hitchhike the signalling molecules and their receptors of the innate immune system to support migration, metastasis and invasion [72]. In general, repair of tissue injury involves enhanced cell proliferation and the activation of a multifactorial network of chemical signals and an inflammatory response to heal the afflicted tissue. Altered, malignant cells proliferate and thrive in such a microenvironment rich in inflammatory cells and growth/survival factors that support their growth [72]. Furthermore, injured, inflamed areas are characterized by superfluous blood flow, chemical signalling for cell proliferation and access to an oversupply of biosynthetic building blocks, clearly providing a permissive resource-rich environment for colonizing tumour cells. Since blood vessels, the suppliers of nutrients and cleaners of metabolites are critically important for cancer cell development, tumours remain limited in size and will not become clinically significant in the absence of angiogenesis [51].

The Ecology of Cancer at the Organism's Scale

Malignant cells, even in early developmental stages (e.g. dysplasia, cells with microscopic characteristics of cancer cells), are known to be extremely prevalent in host tissues, appearing across the lifespan in all multicellular organisms [73, 74]. Unlike microbiota and pathogens/parasites, malignant cells are typically not transmitted between host individuals (but see [12, 22]), though similar to host-pathogen interactions, host genetic and phenotypic traits can influence malignant cell dynamics. The tug of war between malignant cells and their host can lead to evolutionary escalations and "vicious cycles" similar to those observed in certain host-parasite interactions [21]. Thus, cancer cells inevitably have effects beyond the "infected" host organism, by influencing host populations and their ecosystem dynamics through organismal responses to environmental and anthropogenic challenges (e.g. predation, intra- and interspecific competition, parasite infections, pollution, etc.) [75].

The reciprocal ecological and evolutionary interactions between malignant cells and their hosts have previously been considered as oncogenic "noise" and were consequently ignored by evolutionary and ecological researchers. This is an unfortunate oversight since, akin to parasites; malignant cells depend on their hosts for sustenance and proliferation and exploit the host for energy and resources, thereby impairing host health and fitness. Thus, individuals that are able to prevent/minimize malignant cell development, growth and progression have a distinct selective advantage over those exposed to unregulated cancer cells. Consequently, both natural and sexual selection should favour adaptations that limit oncogenic progression and the concomitant reduction in host fitness [76].

Indeed, complex multicellular organisms have evolved numerous control mechanisms at the level of tissue organization (e.g. cell-intrinsic checkpoints), as well as at the organism level such as shifts in behaviour (e.g. reduced activity to conserve energy [77]), shifts in resource allocations (e.g. increased allocation to immune function relative to somatic maintenance [78]), shifts in life history traits (e.g. early onset of reproduction in an attempt to overcome the fitness reducing effect of malignant cells [76]) and shifts in mate choice and mating preferences (e.g. to protect the next generations from malignant cells) [75, 79].

While non-transmissible cancer cells are evolving in response to a novel host environment at each "infection", the host responds to the malignant cells following "pre-arranged", i.e. immunological responses. However, consistent, recurrent exposure to malignant transformations (that appear independently in each generation, since non-transmissible cancer cells perish with the death of the host) will ultimately evoke transgenerational adaptive responses from the host organism [80]. Consequently, theory postulates that malignant cells have been influencing organismal life history traits and strategies over evolutionary time [81].

There are numerous ways for organisms to decrease the impact of cancer, i.e. (i) behavioural adjustments to reduce exposure to carcinogens, or to alleviate the impact of malignant transformations, and (ii) life history trait adjustments to increase fitness even despite of having cancer (reviewed in [75]).

Behavioural Adaptations and Cancer

It is expected that due to the selective pressure of pathogens, including malignant cells, the host should first avoid the source of pathology (prophylactic behaviour), then, if avoidance is unattainable, prevent pathogen progression (evolved tumour-suppressive strategies) and finally, if lethal development is not preventable, alleviate the fitness costs associated with the disease (post-cancer behaviour).

One of the simplest ways to lessen the fitness reducing impact of cancer is to decrease the individual's exposure to the source that may contribute to cancer initiation and development. Habitat selection, such as observed in birds in the Chernobyl area, could result in reduction of carcinogenic radiation encountered from both anthropogenic and natural sources [82]. Following the nuclear catastrophe in Chernobyl in 1986, birds have been observed to breed in sites with the lowest radioactivity [83]. Some fish and aquatic invertebrate species are similarly able to detect heavily polluted areas and avoid sediments contaminated with cancer-causing polycyclic aromatic hydrocarbons (PAH) [84–86].

Although rare, contagious cancers such as the Tasmanian devil facial tumour disease (DFTD) and the canine transmissible venereal tumour (CTVT) provide unique opportunities to study behavioural adaptations to cancer. Tasmanian devil facial tumour disease (DFTD) is transmitted among devils (*Sarcophilus harrisii*) via biting during social interactions, while CTVT is a sexually transmitted clonal cell line of dogs (reviewed in [12]). While DFTD directly impacts survival rate in Tasmanian devils, reducing life expectancy to 6 months following tumour appearance, CTVT mostly impacts individual fitness by affecting the sexual intercourse of dogs (reviewed in [22]). Due to the significant reduction of devil and dog fitness, natural selection should favour individuals capable of discriminating between infectious and noninfectious conspecifics and hence reduce the spread of the diseases. However, as both DFTD and CTVT are transmitted during sexual encounters [87, 88], such an adaptive strategy would also significantly reduce mating opportunities with concomitant fitness reductions. Moreover, DFTD is also transmitted during fights over prey such as roadkill, which further increases the risk of disease transmission [87, 89]. Therefore, conspecific avoidance strategies may result in a very complex evolutionary scenario where natural selection favours less aggressive individuals, while sexual selection favours more aggressive, dominant animals and higher contact rates. The study by Wells et al. [88] indeed has shown that due to their dominant and more aggressive behaviour, infected devils have higher lifetime reproductive success compared to noninfected devils. However, depending on the trade-off between avoiding infected individuals and reduced reproductive success, a less aggressive behaviour in both sexual and feeding encounters could become fixed and form an evolutionary stable strategy (ESS sensu [90]) (reviewed in [91]).

Similar to clonally transmissible cancers, a prophylactic avoidance behaviour may provide fitness advantage in organisms affected by oncogenic pathogens [92]. For example, fibropapillomas (caused by a sexually transmitted herpes virus) invoke significant visible symptoms on green sea turtles (*Chelonia mydas*). The appearance of multiple external epithelial tumours is clear indicators of disease status, giving the opportunity to individuals to avoid affected conspecifics [93].

Apart from alteration of social interactions in response to cancer, changes of individual actions and behaviour may also contribute to strategies to reduce the fitness cost of cancer. For example, consuming antioxidants that potentially counteract the accumulation of cancer-causing DNA mutations may also be a behavioural adaptation to control cancer development [23]. Antioxidants, like carotenoids, can encapsulate free radicals, hence mitigating damage to DNA sequences [94]. Furthermore, changes in diet [77] and self-medication against parasites (potentially including the oncobiont) [3], which is now well known in the animal kingdom as a defence against parasites [95], may have been selected to slow down tumour progression. For example, great apes are known to ingest different plants to decrease intestinal parasite loads [96], and these leaves may also have effective cancer treatment properties (reviewed in [23]). Increasing sleep duration has also been associated with a stronger immune system [97], lower levels of parasitic infections [98] and the production of different hormones that are considered important antitumour agents [99]. Extended sleep time therefore may have a selective advantage that contributes to cancer prevention (reviewed in [23, 75]). Finally, parental behaviour that reduces cancer risks for offspring (e.g. preference for breeding habitats with low mutagen exposure) will also most likely be under positive selection, indicating that adaptive behaviour to cancer avoidance could be a transgenerational process. Another potential scenario is when individuals avoid partners with genetic vulnerabilities and cancer to provide their progeny with superior genetic background ("good genes" hypothesis [100]) or to avoid mating with partners that are unable to provide high-quality parental care ("efficient parent hypothesis" [101]).

Life History (LH) Trait Adjustments to Cancer

Cancer can be thought of as a developing species that behaves in a manner akin to parasites [102]: malignant cells depend on their hosts for sustenance and proliferation, thereby impairing host health and fitness. Direct costs resulting from exploiting the host for resources and energy can cause interindividual (or interpopulation) variation in LH traits such as fecundity and survival [103]. Hosts unable to resist infection by other means (e.g. immunological defences and resistance or long-distance migration) may be able to compensate the parasite/cancer-induced effects by reproducing at an earlier age [104]. Infected individuals have been shown to increase their reproductive activities before dying or being castrated by parasites [105–108] or increase their fitness via kin selection [109, 110]. The most recent example of cancer adjusting reproductive strategies shows that cancerous female *Drosophila* reaches the peak of oviposition earlier in life than healthy females [76]. Transmissible cancers provide one of the best examples of altered life history strategies in response to exposure to cancer. Following the appearance of DFTD, devils have responded to the cancer-induced mortality by rapidly transitioning from a late maturing iteroparous (multiple reproductive cycles) to an early maturing semelparous (single breeding) reproductive strategy [111]. The shift in reaching sexual maturity at an earlier age has most likely been facilitated by increased availability of quality maternal dens as well as increased prey availability brought on by DFTD decimating devil numbers [111]. The latter being supported by the fact that when devil numbers decline the growth rate of subadults increases [112].

The Ecology of Cancer at the Macro-Ecosystem Scale

The impact of cancer on individual fitness will have concomitant implications for ecological interactions, for the structuring of animal communities and ultimately for global biodiversity. For example, similar to other pathogens, individuals with high cancer burden may be subjected to increased predation, a phenomenon that could be exacerbated if predators use cues to detect cancerous prey (e.g. odour differences in healthy and cancerous mice [113]). Competition for abiotic resources and for partners and resisting infectious diseases also represent ecological pressure comparable to predators since they are major causes of mortality and morbidity and ultimately fitness in wildlife [114]. The pressure from infectious diseases could be exacerbated if individuals are immunosuppressed, increasing the probability of becoming infected. Tumours or host responses to the presence of a tumour can trigger immunosuppression [115], and hence individuals affected by cancer generally suffer from a higher vulnerability to infections [93, 116, 117]. Hosts in poor condition are generally more susceptible to pathogen burden and infection intensity, further weakening host condition [118] as well as increasing cancer probability. In wildlife, where cancer is initiated by infections, e.g. otarine herpesvirus-1 infections underlie carcinoma formation in California sea lions (*Zalophus californianus*; [119]), such reciprocal interactions can result in vicious cycles [20, 120, 121].

Unfortunately, documentation of the ecological impact of cancers in general (including transmissible ones) is rare. However, similar to infectious diseases, cancers may have a significant ecological impact on trophic cascades, niche allocation, host-parasite dynamics and disease epidemiology of the ecosystem occupied by the affected host species [21–23]. For example, Tasmanian devil, the world's largest extant marsupial carnivore, is the apex predator on the island of Tasmania. Three additional predators, such as the native marsupial spotted-tailed quoll (*Dasyurus maculatus*), the introduced feral cat (*Felis catus*) and the significantly smaller meso-predator eastern quoll (*Dasyurus viverrinus*) [122, 123], occupy the Tasmanian carnivore guild. With DFTD decimating devil numbers, the number of feral cats has significantly increased. The number of the smaller predators such as the eastern quolls has declined in parallel with the decline in devil numbers indicating devils have provided indirect benefits to the eastern quolls [123]. The negative effects of the transmissible cancer on devil numbers thus appear to have significantly impacted the Tasmanian ecosystem [124, 125].

Anthropogenic Impacts on Cancer Ecology

As discussed above, phenotypic alterations in hosts harbouring malignant cell populations are likely to influence key ecological variables – competitive abilities, feeding strategies, metabolism, immune competence, vulnerability to predators and ability to disperse – in just the same ways as we would expect pathogens to affect these processes [3]. These indirect effects on ecosystems and their potential evolutionary feedbacks (i.e. host biology is shaped by oncogenic processes) are presently poorly understood [3, 75]. The cumulative effect of anthropogenic perturbations on habitat and climate may, however, ultimately result in an upsurge in cancer prevalence in wildlife, further reducing the survival of already endangered species [20, 126].

Humans have recently been declared to be an oncogenic species, with an impact on the environment that causes cancer in other wild populations [127]. Human activities are not only generating environments that are heavily contaminated with anthropogenic chemicals but might also influence cancer rates in the wild through additional processes such as (i) light pollution, (ii) accidental (e.g. human waste) or intentional (e.g. bird feeders) wildlife feeding, (iii) reduction of genetic diversity and/or (iv) modifications of the population dynamics of oncogenic pathogens in human-impacted habitats (reviewed in [127]).

Can Ecological and Evolutionary Sciences Inspire Cancer Therapies?

The true war against cancer did not start when the US president Richard Nixon declared it in 1971 but, more than half a billion years ago, when the first multicellular organisms were confronted with the negative effects of selfish cancerous cells [128]. Natural selection has therefore favoured various adaptations that maximize organismal fitness when subjected to cancerous cell [129]. However, natural selection operates to maximize reproduction and not survival per se, resulting in an increased prevalence of malignant progression in older organisms [78, 130]. As described above, selection may therefore favour increased/earlier reproductive effort to attenuate the fitness cost of cancer [76, 131].

In humans, natural defences against cancer have evolved when life expectancy was short and exposure to mutagenic substances was low. Human life expectancy is presently much longer, and exposure to mutagenic substances is much higher than in the past [132]. Since these changes occurred relatively recently, while evolutionary processes are slow, our natural defences are not in accordance with these novel conditions. These mismatches are basically the main evolutionary reasons for why cancers are becoming more prevalent and a leading cause of mortality worldwide. Consequently, we urgently need to develop innovative therapies against malignant cell proliferation.

Ecological and evolutionary sciences are able to explain the origin and the current resurgence of cancer, but are they also applicable to developing novel therapies? The answer is yes, the most promising example undoubtedly being adaptive therapy [133], whose logic relies on ecological and evolutionary principles. For example, it is well known that chemotherapy frequently produces cancer remission for only a limited period of time, due to intrinsic or acquired resistance to treatment, and hence relapse is often the terminal outcome [134]. The goal is thus to prevent or slow the proliferation of resistant malignant cell populations, since it is these cells that ultimately cause human fatalities [8]. Rather than using therapy aiming at killing the maximum number of malignant cells, the objective of adaptive therapy is to enforce a stable tumour burden by permitting a significant population of chemosensitive cells to survive (Fig. 12.1). In so doing, chemosensitive cells can outcompete

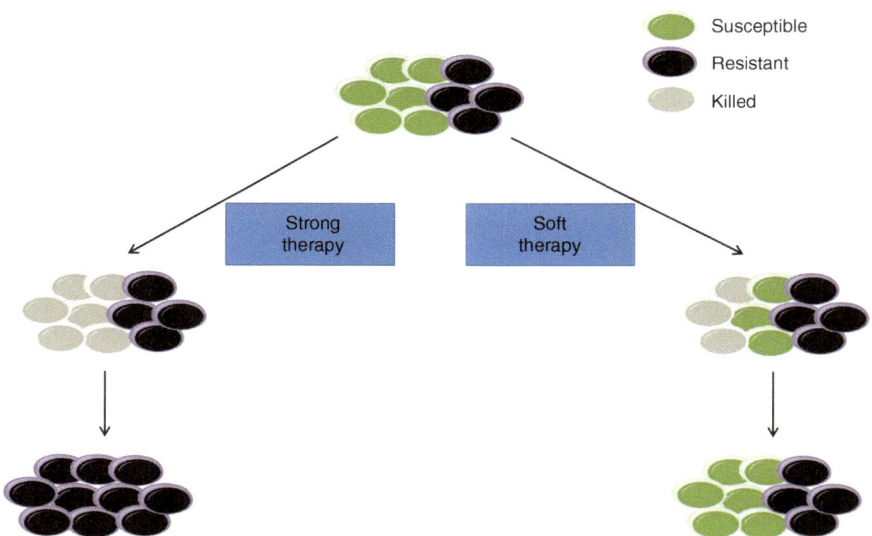

Fig. 12.1 Adaptive therapy principle. Strong chemotherapies eradicate all sensitive cells and hence indirectly favour resistant ones. Conversely, soft chemotherapies kill only a proportion of sensitive cells, so that competition between sensitive and resistant cells is maintained and the tumour size remains constant

chemoresistant subpopulations, hence limiting their expansion. Since acquisition of chemoresistance generally results in impaired cellular fitness as a trade-off (due to the "cost" of phenotypic resistance [13, 78]), therefore these cells are disadvantaged in cell competition. Not only computer simulations show that this strategy results in prolonged survival compared to classical therapies, but in vivo experiments with additional potential side benefits, like lower drug dosage required, are also emerging [133]. Even if significant work remains to be conducted before adaptive therapy becomes a routine cancer treatment option, this approach could potentially be the best compromise to maximize survival in cancer patients when the evolution of drug resistance is unavoidable [135, 136]. When "treatment to kill" is not possible for the metastatic disease, the goal should be to "treat to contain" in a manner that keeps the tumour burden below the level that threatens loss of life or even quality of life. Adaptive therapy illustrates that progression-free survival can be prolonged by integrating evolutionary principles into clinical cancer treatment protocols.

It is well established that oncogenic processes are omnipresent in the body of multicellular organisms and that increasing age results in increasing number of malignant cells [73, 74]. Therefore, the true challenge is not to detect malignant cells per se but to predict which ones will potentially evolve into invasive cancers. Ecologists and evolutionary biologists, in close collaboration with oncologists, have defined an Eco-Evo Index allowing the prediction of tumour evolutionary dynamics [137]. The ecological index considers (i) parameters of the tumour habitat that can be positive (i.e. angiogenesis) or negative (immune cells) to malignant growth and (ii) tumour heterogeneity and the temporal dynamics of this heterogeneity, since these two factors constitute the substrate allowing oncogenic selection to shape tumour evolution. With these two indexes, Maley et al. defined 16 tumour types. The most dangerous being named "rainforest", which corresponds to tumours with high genetic variability, rapid turnover, strong irrigation by blood vessels and high levels of immune predation (which rapidly favours invisible variants). Conversely, the less dangerous tumour type, named "desert", corresponds to tumours with poor variability, low level of angiogenesis and slow turnover. The Eco-Evo Index should soon be routinely applied by oncologists, in addition to other tumour descriptors.

From an evolutionary perspective, cancer is problematic for human health mainly because it often evolves so fast that it is able to outrun our defence systems. In this context, therapies that would decrease the variability of malignant cells would also prevent tumours from reaching their evolutionary potential and would thus reduce their rate of evolution. By reducing cancer evolution rate by two- or threefold, most of our tumours would become harmless beacuse they would go so slow that they would appear beyond our present life expectancy. There are different ways to modify the evolutionary rate of cancer, including alterations in the parameters of tumour microenvironment. In contrast, another strategy is to enhance genetic instability of tumours as it is likely to produce damages to genomic regions that are crucial for their malignancy. Said differently, the level of genetic instability in malignant cells is adjusted by selection to be optimal but not maximal [138], else it would also be detrimental for malignant cell functioning. Enhancing genetic instability could therefore lead tumours to genetic collapse. Although different, the objective of both strategies is to reduce the evolution rate of cancer to become so slow that the malignancy will not have any detrimental impacts before we die from other factors related to senescence.

Numerous therapies against cancer suggest to target driver mutations, because it is indeed those mutations that are frequently responsible for tumour growth. As raised by Gatenby and colleagues [139], the problem with this approach is that sooner or later, malignant cells possessing these driver mutations will become resistant and/or other driver mutations will be favoured. By instead targeting genes critical for malignant functioning to ensure that genes are unable to mutate, will most likely produce dramatic and irreversible damages to the malignant tumours.

We know that cancer dynamics and progression strongly rely on few specific mutations, for example, those occurring on the TP53 gene, and only 350 genes have been identified to contribute to cancer development, i.e. only 1.6% of 20,000 human protein-coding genes [140]. Finding ways to adjust these mutations, and reboot them, would theoretically permit the reactivation of natural defences like apoptosis [141, 142]. Similarly, according to DeGregori [143], cancer is mostly due to the fact that oncogenic mutations are favoured in disturbed microhabitats such as tissues altered by ageing processes/senescence. Restoring conditions that are unfavourable to oncogenic mutations would reduce their selective advantage and hence prevent malignant progression [143]. Importantly, by altering parameters, such oxygen supply has been shown to both inhibit metastasis via endothelial normalization and also to augment metastasis/chemotherapy resistance in ovarian cancer [144, 145].

As discussed above, cancer is a form of parasitic life that for its existence and growth relies on the cooperation of healthy cells in its microenvironment. In the same ways that numerous parasites are able to manipulate species [146], there is also multiple evidence that malignant cells are able to manipulate healthy cells, in a way that is favourable to the tumours [147]. Cancer is hard to cure mostly because of the huge variability of malignant cells that are present inside tumours. However collaborative healthy cells are unlikely to be so variable and should therefore be easier to destroy. By preventing cancer from benefitting of a network of healthy collaborative cells, malignant cells could be constrained to become self-sufficient, which should strongly limit their proliferative potential.

Understanding the metastatic process, from the causes of initiation to factors determining its evolution, is crucial because 90% of cancer-related deaths are due to metastasis. Consequently, it is crucial to elucidate the underpinnings why some cancer cells "decide" to leave their original habitat to become established elsewhere. If this "migration" is due to adverse local conditions, like hypoxia, acidity, lack of space and/or nutrients [148–151], therapies providing primary tumour cells with favourable conditions could theoretically halt the metastatic cascade, even if it is not of course in itself a complete and definitive treatment. From an ecological perspective, regular supplies of small resources could a priori favour a sedentary behaviour of malignant cells (i.e. just by making the cost of leaving higher than staying) without leading to voluminous tumours. The only way to investigate the efficacy of such a treatment would be to conduct experimental analyses on laboratory animals.

It is also crucial to determine the extent to which the level of relatedness between malignant cells is involved in their dispersal behaviour. For instance, in many animal species, dispersal occurs to avoid competition between related individuals [152, 153]. Malignant cells surviving therapies often share similar attributes (e.g. resistance) and are potentially closely related. Since therapies also create damages in the malignant cells' microenvironment, the ultimate consequence of such treatment may be increased local competition between related cells, which ultimately may perpetuate a metastatic behaviour.

Presently therapies that target metastases are often based on decisions on the tumour of origin, and not by considering the novel habitat colonized [154]. For example, bone metastases that originated from prostate cancer and brain metastases originating from breast cancer are still currently treated like prostate and breast cancer. However, the very few migrating cells that succeed in establishing themselves in another tissue (less than 1%) consist of cells that display preadaptations to the novel habitat [155]. Moreover, metastases originating from different primary tumours share similar phenotypic traits (i.e. ecological and evolutionary convergences), but they are not representative of the majority of cells living in the primary tumours. It is therefore unlikely that such metastatic cells can be efficiently eradicated by the same treatment as the one applied to primary tumours.

Tumour heterogeneity is not only caused by the genetic variation of its malignant cells but also by the large diversity of relationships among these cells, such as ability to cooperate and also in differences in competitive and parasitic abilities [156]. Significant tumour growth results from the net result of all such among cellular interactions. Improving our knowledge on the ecological contexts that favour the different types of interactions could in theory permit to exacerbate interactions that are detrimental to tumour growth.

Similarly, conservation biology studies of endangered species could be instructive to understand the ecological and evolutionary contexts that lead to extinction.

In a recent study, Walther et al. [157] suggested that factors involved in species extinction may provide knowledge to improve therapies aimed at reducing the detrimental effects of malignant cells. For example, factors that have been involved in species extinction such as low genetic diversity, low dispersal capacity, long generation time and small geographical distribution have direct parallels to some cancers, i.e. low tumour heterogeneity, reduced metastatic capacity, slow cellular turnover and narrow anatomical range which may provide additional approaches aimed at eradicating cancer cells.

Because resources are often limited, evolutionary theory predicts that any investment in one function is often traded against other functions. Malignant cells are not an exception, and identifying the trade-offs that govern their biology appears as a promising research direction to determine which combinations of treatments may result in their demise [13]. Moreover, biological controls have demonstrated multiple times that the use of combination of different kinds of approaches can be very efficient to control pest species [157]. Similarly, malignant cells resistant to chemotherapies could potentially be treated by the use of oncolytic viruses and/or immunotherapies [13, 158]. Recently, however, a very original and novel therapeutic direction is the use of "ersatzdroges", non-chemotherapy drugs to treat resistant malignant cells [159]. Malignant cells that are chemotherapy and multidrug-resistant have been shown to upregulate the ABCB1 pump (ABC proteins transport various molecules across extra- and intracellular membranes). The nontoxic chemotherapy drug substitutes "ersatzdroges" act as pump substrate and block drug expulsion, resulting in significant reduction in malignant cell proliferation rates. This study strongly suggests that the "ersatzdroges" increased the energy expenditure of the resistant cells and led to decreased fitness [159].

Finally, we must keep in mind the decisive advantage we have over malignant cells. That is, while these cells are governed by natural selection which has no long-term agenda, humans can develop therapies with long-term objectives. Using evolutionary biology will provide us with novel tools to control and eventually cure and hence win the war on cancer.

Acknowledgements This work was supported by an Eric Guiler Tasmanian Devil Research Grants through the Save the Tasmanian devil Appeal of the University of Tasmania Foundation, an Australian Academy of Science, FASIC Early Career Fellowship to BU, an International Associated Laboratory Project France/Australia to FT & BU and a Deakin Faculty of Science Engineering & Built Environment Research Grant Scheme 2017 (SEBE-RGS17-UJVARI). NR is supported by a Holsworth Wildlife Research Endowment. FT is also supported by the ANR EVOCAN, André Hoffmann and la Fondation MAVA. We are grateful to Prof Thomas Madsen for his valuable comments on our manuscript.

References

1. Thomas F, Guegan JF, Renaud F. Ecology and evolution of parasitism. Oxford: Oxford University Press; 2008.
2. Blanchet S, Thomas F, Loot G. Reciprocal effects between host phenotype and pathogens: new insights from an old problem. Trends Parasitol. 2009;25(8):364–9.
3. Thomas F, Jacqueline C, Tissot T, Henard M, Blanchet S, Loot G, et al. The importance of cancer cells for animal evolutionary ecology. Nat Ecol Evol. 2017;1(11):1592–5.
4. Domazet-Loso T, Tautz D. Phylostratigraphic tracking of cancer genes suggests a link to the emergence of multicellularity in metazoa. BMC Biol. 2010;8(1):66.
5. Maynard Smith J, Szathmáry E. The major transitions in evolution. New York: Oxford University Press; 1995.
6. Ratcliff WC, Denison RF, Borrello M, Travisano M. Experimental evolution of multicellularity. Proc Natl Acad Sci U S A. 2012;109(5):1595–600.
7. Leroi AM, Koufopanou V, Burt A. Cancer selection. Nat Rev Cancer. 2003;3(3):226–31.
8. Greaves M, Maley CC. Clonal evolution in cancer. Nature. 2012;481(7381):306–13.
9. Nowell P. The clonal evolution of tumor cell populations. Science. 1976;194(4260):23–8.
10. Merlo L, Pepper J, Reid B, Maley C. Cancer as an evolutionary and ecological process. Nat Rev Cancer. 2006;6:924–35.
11. Podlaha O, Riester M, De S, Michor F. Evolution of the cancer genome. Trends Genet. 2012;28(4):155–63.
12. Ujvari B, Gatenby RA, Thomas F. Transmissible cancer, the evolution of inter-individual metastasis. In: Ujvari B, Roche B, Thomas F, editors. Ecology and evolution of cancer. London: Elsevier; 2017. p. 290.

13. Aktipis CA, Boddy AM, Gatenby RA, Brown JS, Maley CC. Life history trade-offs in cancer evolution. Nat Rev Cancer. 2013;13(12):883–92.
14. Korolev KS, Xavier JB, Gore J. Turning ecology and evolution against cancer. Nat Rev Cancer. 2014;14(5):371–80.
15. Robert J. Comparative study of tumorigenesis and tumor immunity in invertebrates and non-mammalian vertebrates. Dev Comp Immunol. 2010;34(9):915–25.
16. Scharrer B, Lochhead MS. Tumors in the invertebrates: a review. Cancer Res. 1950;10:403–19.
17. Nagy JD, Victor EM, Cropper JH. Why don't all whales have cancer? A novel hypothesis resolving Peto's paradox. Integr Comp Biol. 2007;47(2):317–28.
18. Schlumberger HG, Lucké B. Tumors of fishes, amphibians and reptiles. Cancer Res. 1948;8:657–754.
19. Maden D. Reptile medicine and surgery. 2nd ed. St Louis: Saunders; 2005. 1264 p.
20. Madsen T, Arnal A, Vittecoq M, Bernex F, Abadie J, Labrut S, et al. Chapter 2 – Cancer prevalence and etiology in wild and captive animals. In: Ecology and evolution of cancer. London: Academic; 2017. p. 11–46.
21. Ujvari B, Beckmann C, Biro PA, Arnal A, Tasiemski A, Massol F, et al. Cancer and life-history traits: lessons from host-parasite interactions. Parasitology. 2016;143(5):533–41.
22. Ujvari B, Gatenby RA, Thomas F. The evolutionary ecology of transmissible cancers. Infect Genet Evol. 2016;39:293–303.
23. Vittecoq M, Ducasse H, Arnal A, Møller AP, Ujvari B, Jacqueline CB, et al. Animal behaviour and cancer. Anim Behav. 2015;101(0):19–26.
24. Gatenby RA, Gillies RJ. A microenvironmental model of carcinogenesis. Nat Rev Cancer. 2008;8(1):56–61.
25. Ujvari B, Papenfuss AT, Belov K. Transmissible cancers in an evolutionary context. Inside Cell. 2015;1(1):1–10.
26. Nguyen DX, Bos PD, Massagué J. Metastasis: from dissemination to organ-specific colonization. Nat Rev Cancer. 2009;9(4):274–84.
27. Hanahan D, Weinberg RA. Hallmarks of cancer: the next generation. Cell. 2011;144(5):646–74.
28. Ehrlich PR. Which animal will invade? In: Mooney HA, Drake JA, editors. Ecology of biological invasions of North America and Hawaii. New York: Springer; 1984. p. 79–95.
29. Lodge DM. Biological invasions: lessons for ecology. Trends Ecol Evol. 1993;8(4):133–7.
30. Sakai AK, Allendorf FW, Holt JS, Lodge DM, Molofsky J, With KA, et al. The population biology of invasive species. Annu Rev Ecol Syst. 2001;32(1):305–32.
31. Lowry E, Rollinson EJ, Laybourn AJ, Scott TE, Aiello-Lammens ME, Gray SM, et al. Biological invasions: a field synopsis, systematic review, and database of the literature. Ecol Evol. 2013;3(1):182–96.
32. Kolar CS, Lodge DM. Progress in invasion biology: predicting invaders. Trends Ecol Evol. 2001;16(4):199–204.
33. Reznick D, Bryant MJ, Bashey F. r- and K-selection revisited: the role of population regulation in life-history evolution. Ecology. 2002;83(6):1509–20.
34. Lockwood JL, Cassey P, Blackburn T. The role of propagule pressure in explaining species invasions. Trends Ecol Evol. 2005;20(5):223–8.
35. Schlichting CD, Levin DA. Phenotypic plasticity: an evolving plant character. Biol J Linn Soc. 1986;29(1):37–47.
36. Davidson AM, Jennions M, Nicotra AB. Do invasive species show higher phenotypic plasticity than native species and, if so, is it adaptive? A meta-analysis. Ecol Lett. 2011;14(4):419–31.
37. Gatenby RA, Gillies RJ, Brown JS. Of cancer and cave fish. Nat Rev Cancer. 2011;11(4):237–8.
38. Lujambio A, Esteller M. How epigenetics can explain human metastasis: a new role for microRNAs. Cell Cycle. 2009;8(3):377–82.
39. Rodenhiser D. Epigenetic contributions to cancer metastasis. Clin Exp Metastasis. 2009;26(1):5–18.
40. Ardura A, Zaiko A, Morán P, Planes S, Garcia-Vazquez E. Epigenetic signatures of invasive status in populations of marine invertebrates. Sci Rep. 2017;7:42193.

41. Jaenisch R, Bird A. Epigenetic regulation of gene expression: how the genome integrates intrinsic and environmental signals. Nat Genet. 2003;33 Suppl:245–54.
42. Bird A. Perceptions of epigenetics. Nature. 2007;447(7143):396–8.
43. Seftor REB, Seftor EA, Postovit L-M, Hendrix MJC. Overview of tumor cells and the microenvironment. In: Leong SPL, editor. From local invasion to metastatic cancer: involvement of distant sites through the lymphovascular system. Totowa: Humana Press; 2009. p. 69–73.
44. Polyak K, Haviv I, Campbell IG. Co-evolution of tumor cells and their microenvironment. Trends Genet. 2009;25(1):30–8.
45. Bhowmick NA, Neilson EG, Moses HL. Stromal fibroblasts in cancer initiation and progression. Nature. 2004;432(7015):332–7.
46. Hu M, Polyak K. Microenvironmental regulation of cancer development. Curr Opin Genet Dev. 2008;18(1):27–34.
47. Nelson CM, Bissell MJ. Of extracellular matrix, scaffolds, and signaling: tissue architecture regulates development, homeostasis, and cancer. Annu Rev Cell Dev Biol. 2006;22(1):287–309.
48. Orimo A, Weinberg RA. Stromal fibroblasts in cancer: a novel tumor-promoting cell type. Cell Cycle. 2006;5(15):1597–601.
49. Tlsty TD, Coussens LM. Tumor stroma and regulation of cancer development. Ann Rev Pathol Mech Dis. 2006;1(1):119–50.
50. Lorenzo P, Hussain MI, González L. Role of allelopathy during invasion process by alien invasive plants in terrestrial ecosystems. In: Cheema ZA, Farooq M, Wahid A, editors. Allelopathy. Berlin/Heidelberg: Springer; 2013. p. 3–21.
51. Alfarouk KO, Ibrahim ME, Gatenby RA, Brown JS. Riparian ecosystems in human cancers. Evol Appl. 2013;6(1):46–53.
52. Warburg O. Ueber den stoffwechsel der tumoren. London: Constable; 1930.
53. Hsu PP, Sabatini DM. Cancer cell metabolism: Warburg and beyond. Cell. 2008;134(5):703–7.
54. Hans HK, Taeho K, Euiyong K, Ji Kyoung P, Seok-Ju P, Hyun J, et al. The mitochondrial Warburg effect: a cancer enigma. IBC. 2009;1:7.
55. Najafov A, Alessi DR. Uncoupling the Warburg effect from cancer. Proc Natl Acad Sci U S A. 2010;107(45):19135–6.
56. Vander Heiden MG, Cantley LC, Thompson CB. Understanding the Warburg effect: the metabolic requirements of cell proliferation. Science. 2009;324(5930):1029–33.
57. Pfeiffer T, Schuster S, Bonhoeffer S. Cooperation and competition in the evolution of ATP-producing pathways. Science. 2001;292(5516):504–7.
58. Gatenby RA, Gillies RJ. Why do cancers have high aerobic glycolysis? Nat Rev Cancer. 2004;4(11):891–9.
59. Gravenmier CA, Siddique M, Gatenby RA. Adaptation to stochastic temporal variations in intratumoral blood flow: the Warburg effect as a bet hedging strategy. Bull Math Biol. 2018;80(5):954–70.
60. Epstein T, Gatenby RA, Brown JS. The Warburg effect as an adaptation of cancer cells to rapid fluctuations in energy demand. PLoS One. 2017;12(9):e0185085.
61. Huber V, De Milito A, Harguindey S, Reshkin SJ, Wahl ML, Rauch C, et al. Proton dynamics in cancer. J Transl Med. 2010;8:57.
62. Gabrilovich DI, Nagaraj S. Myeloid-derived-suppressor cells as regulators of the immune system. Nat Rev Immunol. 2009;9(3):162–74.
63. Murdoch C, Muthana M, Coffelt SB, Lewis CE. The role of myeloid cells in the promotion of tumour angiogenesis. Nat Rev Cancer. 2008;8(8):618–31.
64. Gatenby RA, Gawlinski ET. A reaction-diffusion model of cancer invasion. Cancer Res. 1996;56(24):5745–53.
65. Gatenby RA, Gawlinski ET, Gmitro AF, Kaylor B, Gillies RJ. Acid-mediated tumor invasion: a multidisciplinary study. Cancer Res. 2006;66(10):5216–23.
66. Martínez-Zaguilán R, Seftor EA, Seftor RE, Chu YW, Gillies RJ, Hendrix MJ. Acidic pH enhances the invasive behavior of human melanoma cells. Clin Exp Metastasis. 1996;14(2):176–86.

67. Britton-Simmons KH, Abbott KC. Short- and long-term effects of disturbance and propagule pressure on a biological invasion. J Ecol. 2008;96(1):68–77.
68. Simberloff D. The role of propagule pressure in biological invasions. Annu Rev Ecol Evol Syst. 2009;40(1):81–102.
69. Leung B, Mandrak NE. The risk of establishment of aquatic invasive species: joining invasibility and propagule pressure. Proc R Soc B Biol Sci. 2007;274(1625):2603–9.
70. Ducasse H, Arnal A, Vittecoq M, Daoust Simon P, Ujvari B, Jacqueline C, et al. Cancer: an emergent property of disturbed resource-rich environments? Ecology meets personalized medicine. Evol Appl. 2015;8(6):527–40.
71. Siddle HV, Kaufman J. A tale of two tumours: comparison of the immune escape strategies of contagious cancers. Mol Immunol. 2013;55(2):190–3.
72. Coussens LM, Werb Z. Inflammation and cancer. Nature. 2002;420(6917):860–7.
73. Bissell MJ, Hines WC. Why don't we get more cancer? A proposed role of the microenvironment in restraining cancer progression. Nat Med. 2011;17(3):320–9.
74. Folkman J, Kalluri R. Cancer without disease. Nature. 2004;427(6977):787.
75. Roche B, Møller AP, DeGregori J, Thomas F. Chapter 13 – Cancer in animals: reciprocal feedbacks between evolution of cancer resistance and ecosystem functioning. In: Ecology and evolution of cancer. London: Academic; 2017. p. 181–91.
76. Arnal A, Jacqueline C, Ujvari B, Leger L, Moreno C, Faugere D, et al. Cancer brings forward oviposition in the fly Drosophila melanogaster. Ecol Evol. 2017;7(1):272–6.
77. Thomas F, Rome S, Mery F, Dawson E, Montagne J, Biro Peter A, et al. Changes in diet associated with cancer: an evolutionary perspective. Evol Appl. 2017;10(7):651–7.
78. Jacqueline C, Biro Peter A, Beckmann C, Moller Anders P, Renaud F, Sorci G, et al. Cancer: a disease at the crossroads of trade-offs. Evol Appl. 2016;10(3):215–25.
79. Nunney L. Chapter 1 – the evolutionary origins of cancer and of its control by immune policing and genetic suppression A2 – Ujvari, Beata. In: Roche B, Thomas F, editors. Ecology and evolution of cancer. London: Academic; 2017. p. 1–9.
80. Casás-Selves M, DeGregori J. How cancer shapes evolution, and how evolution shapes cancer. Evolution. 2011;4(4):624–34.
81. Thomas F, Ujvari B, Renaud F, Vincent M. Cancer adaptations: atavism, de novo selection, or something in between? BioEssays. 2017;39(8):1700039.
82. Aarkrog A. Environmental radiation and radioactive releases. Int J Radiat Biol. 1990;57(4):619–31.
83. Møller AP, Mousseau TA. Birds prefer to breed in sites with low radioactivity in Chernobyl. Proc R Soc B Biol Sci. 2007;274(1616):1443.
84. da Luz TN, Ribeiro R, Sousa JP. Avoidance tests with collembola and earthworms as early screening tools for site-specific assessment of polluted soils. Environ Toxicol Chem. 2009;23(9):2188–93.
85. De Lange HJ, Sperber V, Peeters Edwin THM. Avoidance of polycyclic aromatic hydrocarbon–contaminated sediments by the freshwater invertebrates Gammarus pulex and Asellus aquaticus. Environ Toxicol Chem. 2009;25(2):452–7.
86. Giattina JD, Garton RR. A review of the preference-avoidance response of fishes to aquatic contaminants. Residue Rev. 1983;87:43–90.
87. Hamede RK, McCallum H, Jones M. Seasonal, demographic and density-related patterns of contact between Tasmanian devils (Sarcophilus harrisii): implications for transmission of devil facial tumour disease. Austral Ecol. 2008;33(5):614–22.
88. Wells K, Hamede RK, Kerlin DH, Storfer A, Hohenlohe PA, Jones ME, et al. Infection of the fittest: devil facial tumour disease has greatest effect on individuals with highest reproductive output. Ecol Lett. 2017;20(6):770–8.
89. Pemberton D, Renouf D. A field-study of communication and social-behavior of the Tasmanian devil at feeding sites. Aust J Zool. 1993;41(5):507–26.
90. Smith JM, Price GR. The logic of animal conflict. Nature. 1973;246(5427):15–8.

91. Russell T, Madsen T, Thomas F, Raven N, Hamede R, Ujvari B. Oncogenesis as a selective force: adaptive evolution in the face of a transmissible Cancer. BioEssays. 2018;40(3):1700146.

92. zur Hausen H. The search for infectious causes of human cancers: where and why. Virology. 2009;392(1):1–10.

93. Aguirre AA, Lutz PL. Marine turtles as sentinels of ecosystem health: is fibropapillomatosis an Indicator? EcoHealth. 2004;1(3):275–83.

94. Møller AP, Biard C, Blount JD, Houston DC, Ninni P, Saino N, et al. Carotenoid-dependent signals: indicators of foraging efficiency, immunocompetence or detoxification ability? Avian Poultry Biol Rev. 2000;11(3):137–59.

95. de Roode JC, Lefèvre T, Hunter MD. Self-medication in animals. Science. 2013;340(6129):150.

96. Huffman MA. Self-Medicative behavior in the African great apes: an evolutionary perspective into the origins of human traditional medicine. In addition to giving us a deeper understanding of our closest living relatives, the study of great ape self-medication provides a window into the origins of herbal medicine use by humans and promises to provide new insights into ways of treating parasite infections and other serious diseases. Bioscience. 2001;51(8):651–61.

97. Bryant PA, Trinder J, Curtis N. Sick and tired: does sleep have a vital role in the immune system? Nat Rev Immunol. 2004;4(6):457–67.

98. Preston BT, Capellini I, McNamara P, Barton RA, Nunn CL. Parasite resistance and the adaptive significance of sleep. BMC Evol Biol. 2009;9:7.

99. Blask DE. Melatonin, sleep disturbance and cancer risk. Sleep Med Rev. 2009;13(4):257–64.

100. Moller APM, Alatalo RV. Good-genes effects in sexual selection. Proc R Soc B Biol Sci. 1999;266(1414):85.

101. Hoelzer GA. The good parent process of sexual selection. Anim Behav. 1989;38(6):1067–78.

102. Duesberg P, McCormack A. Is carcinogenesis a form of speciation? Cell Cycle. 2011;10:2100–4.

103. Thomas F, Guégan J-F, Michalakis Y, Renaud F. Parasites and host life-history traits: implications for community ecology and species co-existence. Int J Parasitol. 2000;30(5):669–74.

104. Mark RLF. Parasitism and host reproductive effort. Oikos. 1993;67(3):444–50.

105. Adamo SA. Evidence for adaptive changes in egg laying in crickets exposed to bacteria and parasites. Anim Behav. 1999;57(1):117–24.

106. Minchella DJ, Loverde PT. A cost of increased early reproductive effort in the snail Biomphalaria glabrata. Am Nat. 1981;118(6):876–81.

107. Polak M, Starmer WT. Parasite-induced risk of mortality elevates reproductive effort in male Drosophila. Proc R Soc B Biol Sci. 1998;265(1411):2197–201.

108. Sorci G, Clobert J, Michalakis Y. Cost of reproduction and cost of parasitism in the common Lizard, Lacerta vivipara. OIKOS. 1996;76:121–30.

109. Débarre F, Lion S, van Baalen M, Gandon S. Evolution of host life-history traits in a spatially structured host-parasite system. Am Nat. 2012;179(1):52–63.

110. Iritani R, Iwasa Y. Parasite infection drives the evolution of state-dependent dispersal of the host. Theor Popul Biol. 2014;92:1–13.

111. Jones ME, Cockburn A, Hamede R, Hawkins C, Hesterman H, Lachish S, et al. Life-history change in disease-ravaged Tasmanian devil populations. Proc Natl Acad Sci. 2008;105(29):10023–7.

112. Lachish S, McCallum H, Jones M. Demography, disease and the devil: life-history changes in a disease-affected population of Tasmanian devils (Sarcophilus harrisii). J Anim Ecol. 2009;78(2):427–36.

113. Alves GJ, Vismari L, Lazzarini R, Merusse JLB, Palermo-Neto J. Odor cues from tumor-bearing mice induces neuroimmune changes. Behav Brain Res. 2010;214(2):357–67.

114. Scott ME. The impact of infection and disease on animal populations: implications for conservation biology. Conserv Biol. 1988;2(1):40–56.

115. Pollock Raphael E, Roth JA. Cancer-induced immunosuppression: implications for therapy? Semin Surg Oncol. 1989;5(6):414–9.
116. von Bernstorff W, Voss M, Freichel S, Schmid A, Vogel I, Jöhnk C, et al. Systemic and local immunosuppression in pancreatic cancer patients. Cli Cancer Res. 2001;7(3):925s.
117. Kim R, Emi M, Tanabe K. Cancer immunosuppression and autoimmune disease: beyond immunosuppressive networks for tumour immunity. Immunology. 2006;119(2):254–64.
118. Beldomenico PM, Begon M. Disease spread, susceptibility and infection intensity: vicious circles? Trends Ecol Evol. 2010;25(1):21–7.
119. Newman SJ, Smith SA. Marine mammal neoplasia: a review. Vet Pathol. 2006;43(6):865–80.
120. Moller A, Nielsen J. Malaria and risk of predation: A comparative study of birds. Ecology. 2007;88:871–81.
121. Murray D, Cary JR, Keith LB. Interactive effects of sublethal nematodes and nutritional status on snowshoe hare vulnerability to predation; 1997. 250 p.
122. Jones M. Character displacement in Australian dasyurid carnivores: size relationships and prey size patterns. Ecology. 1997;78(8):2569–87.
123. Hollings T, Jones M, Mooney N, McCallum H. Trophic cascades following the disease-induced decline of an apex predator, the tasmanian devil. Conserv Biol. 2014;28(1):63–75.
124. Petchey OL. Species diversity, species extinction, and ecosystem function. Am Nat. 2000;155(5):696–702.
125. Hollings T, Jones M, Mooney N, McCallum H. Disease-induced decline of an apex predator drives invasive dominated states and threatens biodiversity. Ecology. 2016;97(2):394–405.
126. McAloose D, Newton AL. Wildlife cancer: a conservation perspective. Nat Rev Cancer. 2009;9(7):517–26.
127. Giraudeau M, Sepp T, Ujvari B, Ewald PW, Thomas F. Human activities might influence oncogenic processes in wild animal populations. Nat Ecol Evol. 2018;2:1065–70.
128. Aktipis CA, Nesse Randolph M. Evolutionary foundations for cancer biology. Evol Appl. 2013;6(1):144–59.
129. DeGregori J. Evolved tumor suppression: why are we so good at not getting cancer? Cancer Res. 2011;71(11):3739.
130. Hochberg Michael E, Thomas F, Assenat E, Hibner U. Preventive evolutionary medicine of cancers. Evol Appl. 2012;6(1):134–43.
131. Smith KR, Hanson HA, Mineau GP, Buys SS. Effects of BRCA1 and BRCA2 mutations on female fertility. Proc R Soc B Biol Sci. 2012;279(1732):1389–95.
132. Nesse RM, George C. Why we get sick: the new science of Darwinian medicine. New York: Williams Times Books; 1995.
133. Gatenby RA, Silva AS, Gillies RJ, Frieden BR. Adaptive therapy. Cancer Res. 2009;69(11):4894.
134. Holohan C, Van Schaeybroeck S, Longley DB, Johnston PG. Cancer drug resistance: an evolving paradigm. Nat Rev Cancer. 2013;13(10):714–26.
135. Enriquez-Navas PM, Gatenby RA. Chapter 14 – Applying tools from evolutionary biology to cancer research A2 – Ujvari, Beata. In: Roche B, Thomas F, editors. Ecology and evolution of cancer. London: Academic; 2017. p. 193–200.
136. Ledford H. Cancer treatment: the killer within. Nature. 2014;508(7494):24–6.
137. Maley CC, Aktipis A, Graham TA, Sottoriva A, Boddy AM, Janiszewska M, et al. Classifying the evolutionary and ecological features of neoplasms. Nat Rev Cancer. 2017;17:605.
138. Ruchira SD, Gutteridge A, Swanton C, Maley Carlo C, Graham TA. Modelling the evolution of genetic instability during tumour progression. Evol Appl. 2012;6(1):20–33.
139. Gatenby RA, Cunningham JJ, Brown JS. Evolutionary triage governs fitness in driver and passenger mutations and suggests targeting never mutations. Nat Commun. 2014;5:5499.
140. Stratton MR, Campbell PJ, Futreal PA. The cancer genome. Nature. 2009;458:719.
141. Martinez JD. Restoring p53 tumor suppressor activity as an anticancer therapeutic strategy. Future Oncol (London, England). 2010;6(12):1857–62.

142. Acosta J, Wang W, Feldser DM. Off and back-on again: a tumor suppressor's tale. Oncogene. 2018;37:3058.
143. DeGregori J. Adaptive oncogenesis: a new understanding of how cancer evolves inside us. Cambridge, MA: Harvard University Press; 2018.
144. Mazzone M, Dettori D, Leite de Oliveira R, Loges S, Schmidt T, Jonckx B, et al. Heterozygous deficiency of PHD2 restores tumor oxygenation and inhibits metastasis via endothelial normalization. Cell. 2009;136(5):839–51.
145. Dorayappan KDP, Wanner R, Wallbillich JJ, Saini U, Zingarelli R, Suarez AA, et al. Hypoxia-induced exosomes contribute to a more aggressive and chemoresistant ovarian cancer pheno-type: a novel mechanism linking STAT3/Rab proteins. Oncogene. 2018;37:3806.
146. Hughes DP, Brodeur J, Thomas F. Host manipulation by parasites. Oxford University Press; Oxford, UK, 2012.
147. Tissot T, Arnal A, Jacqueline C, Poulin R, Lefèvre T, Mery F, et al. Host manipulation by can-cer cells: expectations, facts, and therapeutic implications. BioEssays. 2016;38(3):276–85.
148. Estrella V, Chen T, Lloyd M, Wojtkowiak J, Cornnell HH, Ibrahim-Hashim A, et al. Acidity generated by the tumor microenvironment drives local invasion. Cancer Res. 2013;73(5):1524.
149. Moellering RE, Black KC, Krishnamurty C, Baggett BK, Stafford P, Rain M, et al. Acid treatment of melanoma cells selects for invasive phenotypes. Clin Exp Metastasis. 2008;25(4):411–25.
150. Orlando P, Gatenby R, Brown J. Tumor evolution in space: the effects of competition coloni-zation tradeoffs on tumor invasion dynamics. Front Oncol. 2013;3:45.
151. Verduzco D, Lloyd M, Xu L, Ibrahim-Hashim A, Balagurunathan Y, Gatenby RA, et al. Intermittent hypoxia selects for genotypes and phenotypes that increase survival, invasion, and therapy resistance. PLoS One. 2015;10(3):e0120958.
152. Bitume EV, Bonte D, Ronce O, Bach F, Flaven E, Olivieri I, et al. Density and genetic related-ness increase dispersal distance in a subsocial organism. Ecol Lett. 2013;16(4):430–7.
153. Ronce O. How does it feel to be like a rolling stone? Ten questions about dispersal evolution. Annu Rev Ecol Evol Syst. 2007;38(1):231–53.
154. Cunningham JJ, Brown JS, Vincent TL, Gatenby RA. Divergent and convergent evolution in metastases suggest treatment strategies based on specific metastatic sites. Evol Med Public Health. 2015;2015(1):76–87.
155. Riethdorf S, Wikman H, Pantel K. Review: biological relevance of disseminated tumor cells in cancer patients. Int J Cancer. 2008;123(9):1991–2006.
156. Tissot T, Ujvari B, Solary E, Lassus P, Roche B, Thomas F. Do cell-autonomous and non-cell-autonomous effects drive the structure of tumor ecosystems? Biochimica et Biophysica Acta (BBA) Rev Cancer. 2016;1865(2):147–54.
157. Walther V, Hiley CT, Shibata D, Swanton C, Turner PE, Maley CC. Can Oncology recapitu-late paleontology? Lessons from species extinctions. Nat Rev Clin Oncol. 2015;12(5):273–85. https://doi.org/10.1038/nrclinonc.2015.12.
158. Gatenby RA, Brown J, Vincent T. Lessons from applied ecology: cancer control using an evolutionary double bind. Cancer Res. 2009;69(19):7499.
159. Kam Y, Das T, Tian H, Foroutan P, Ruiz E, Martinez G, Minton S, Gillies RJ, Gatenby RA. Sweat but no gain: Inhibiting proliferation of multidrug resistant cancer cells with "ersatzdroges". Int J Cancer. 2015;136:E188–96. https://doi.org/10.1002/ijc.29158.

Index